THE METHOD

The
METHOD

The PRACTICAL PATH to LIVING YOUR PURPOSE and POTENTIAL

XO,
Dr. T

DR. TRACY THOMAS

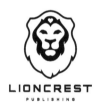

LIONCREST
PUBLISHING

THE METHOD

The Practical Path to Living Your Purpose and Potential

ISBN   978-1-61961-552-6 *Paperback*

978-1-61961-553-3 *Ebook*

978-1-61961-776-6 *Audiobook*

I want to dedicate this book to all the clients I've ever had the privilege of working with, who have entrusted me with their most valuable possession: their intentions for their lives. Most of them, in fact, literally trusted me with their very survival. They have fought and persevered through intense pain and darkness on their way to meeting The Method. They have committed themselves wholeheartedly, shown up to do the work every day, and they continue to apply this methodology at greater and greater levels—even in the face of humbling human moments. Through it all, they've loved me unconditionally.

With these courageous people, I share conversations immersed in unprecedented honesty. Their willingness to bare their souls and confront their shame has shown me a level of humanity I've not experienced anywhere else. They are people who come to play, who take their commitment to The Method seriously, who get up when they fall, who come back asking for more, and who prove this methodology is not only effective when implemented, but also entertaining and fun. They have given me the most mind-blowing, purposeful career I could ever have imagined—the career I've always wanted. Their commitment to The Method has proven to be a gift not only to themselves, but also a gift to me. Our work together allows each of us to be completely who we are, and in so doing, allows us to serve each other's purpose and potential.

Everything my clients invest in themselves helps me to grow my emotional and behavioral training practice. By allowing me to share in their struggles and partner in their growth, they offer a priceless gift to the clients who will come after them.

This book is the direct result of our partnership. We are co-creators, and we share the honor of making this information available to many others who will benefit from it.

Even though I know they may not believe this (because they're still working on believing), they mean as much to me as I mean to them. To use the language of The Method, this book is—in all integrity, honesty, and truth—dedicated to them.

CONTENTS

———

GETTING THE MOST OUT OF THIS BOOK

———

The more you get out of this book, the more you'll experience your full potential each and every day of your life!

In order to get the most out of this book:

1. Develop a deep, driving desire to master the principles of living your purpose and potential in the most simple methodology possible: "The Method."
2. Don't be in a hurry...Take the time to let every part of The Method really sink in. This is a new way of being.
3. Underscore (or highlight) each important idea...treat this book like a guide.
4. Read with the intention of passing on something you learned in each chapter within twenty-four hours.

Know that when your true Self is living its purpose and potential, it connects with others who are doing the same thing.

5. As you read, stop and ask yourself how you can apply each idea. Write in the margins or keep a journal with your insights and action list.

6. Take action—connect to your Self. Apply what you have learned, growing in trust of your internal navigation system, building epic emotional strength, so that you are living in integrity each day.

7. Any moment you're experiencing pain or struggle, review your notes and anything that you've underlined to bring you back to a connection with your Self. Continue to apply what you have learned so that The Method becomes your new normal.

8. Carry this book around with you so that it functions like a handbook that you can refer to anytime, so that you don't miss out on a single day of experiencing your full potential.

9. Join a community of people learning and applying The Method into their life every day. Join our Facebook group, "The Art of Self Control" at the link on the next page, "More Things To Help You."

MORE THINGS
TO HELP YOU

———

Access links (and additional descriptions) for all resources listed here can be found at www.drtracyinc.com/ morethingstohelpyou/

As we add to this growing list of resources over time, you will find those new additions at this link.

1. www.DrTracyInc.com
2. (video series) "Turning Stress Into Success—The 5 Ways Successful Entrepreneurs Use Epic Emotional Strength to Build Their Empires, Their Impact, and Their Income, All While Enjoying Epic Health, Happiness, and Freedom"
3. (video series) "The Six Shifts Strategy to Take Control of Your Behaviors, Your Emotions, and Destiny"

4. (video series) Firsthand Client Accounts of How The Method Transformed Their Life

5. The Art of Self Control: Our Facebook Group: Join a community of people learning and applying The Method into their life every day, we welcome you to join our Facebook group, "The Art of Self Control."

6. Follow Us on Facebook from Anywhere! Follow us on Facebook to get the latest updates and be the first to view videos from Dr. T, as well as gain access to live events.

7. Our YouTube Channel Will Change Your Life: Dr. T is creating content every day that is transforming people's lives. Be plugged in to our YouTube channel so that you too can receive the latest insights directly from Dr. T.

8. You + Dr. T + Instagram = The Perfect Combo On-the-Go! Dr. T is the perfect companion to have on-the-go via your Instagram mobile app. When you're in need of just the right motivational thought, Dr. T will be right with you to deliver that message.

9. Your Daily Transformation Begins With a Steady Diet of 'Dr. T' via Twitter: Whatever your challenge, you can count on Dr. T to give you powerful, straight insight on lasting transformation. Dr. T is your transformational news channel.

10. The Power of Dr. Tracy in over Twenty National Publications: You name it—*Redbook, Men's Health,*

Mind Body Green, Shape, Women's Health, and more—national publications have sought out Dr. T to provide insights and guidance to their readers. We've gathered a cross-section of topics for you to explore.

11. The "Total Life Reset Manual" is the Ultimate Starter Resource: The "Total Life Reset Manual" is the ultimate starter resource for changing the mindsets that are holding you back. The TLR Manual is ALL of Dr. T's seven e-books in one big, affordable bundle. Whether you are struggling to stay fulfilled in your career, ready to strengthen or redefine your relationships, or need help navigating depression, anxiety, or addiction—this workbook contains over twenty-five self-awareness exercises that add up to seven weeks of core mindset changes that will completely reset your life.

12. Individual E-books: Want to dip your toe in the water? The TLR Manual is ALL of Dr. T's seven e-books together. If you'd like to begin by zeroing in on one topic-specific area, please do. You can individually select from the following:

- Redefining Happy and Healthy
- Redefining You
- Redefining Career and Purpose
- Redefining Relationships
- Redefining Anxiety
- Redefining Depression
- Redefining Addiction

13. Go All the Way! If you'd like to comprehensively upgrade the relationship with your Self as well as every relationship in your life, our virtual programs can take you to the next level. While The Method is highly effective when you practice it on your own, if your navigation system is inspiring you to work with Dr. T more directly, then fabulous! Believe me, there's nothing I'd love more than to help you incorporate The Method into your life in the most accelerated way. You can take action now by going to thedrtsolution.com.

14. Emotional Training: While you're at it, why not make Dr. T's ever growing Emotional Training content an integral part of your ongoing life transformation? GREAT NEWS! NOW YOU CAN, at a low monthly fee! Because everyone deserves the emotional training they never experienced growing up, Dr. T is making emotional training affordable for everyone. Dr. T is overflowing with content and is constantly sharing new video and audio emotional strength training modules with her community of followers each week. These powerful trainings help people grow the emotional foundation they need to live their purpose and potential each day. With over 130 hours of emotional training modules and growing, Dr. T is fulfilling her dream to provide easy and accessible emotional training to everyone who needs it. This link will take you to everything you need to know to decide if this next step is right for you: thedrtsolution.com.

FOR THE MEDIA

Dr. T is a licensed clinical psychologist, a behavioral specialist, and a performance coach. She's a recovery strategist/interventionist with over twenty years of expertise in maximizing human performance and potential in both the corporate world and the clinical field. Dr. T is a former corporate trainer for Fortune 100 Companies, a former elite athlete, and an MBA.

She's worked for years with the über-wealthy and professional people from many industries, to alleviate complex emotional and behavioral conditions where others before her had failed. She's helped countless clients transcend their disorders and saved them and their families from a lifetime of pain and lost potential.

As a clinical doctor and a performance coach, she's trained to diagnose and treat clinical disorders as well as facilitate behavioral transformation. Based on the success she's had helping people change their lives, she's also a respected expert for over twenty national magazines and media outlets.

FOR ALL MEDIA INQUIRIES, PLEASE CONTACT: drt@drtracyinc.com

INTRODUCTION

———

There are as many different stories of suffering as there are people in the world. Nevertheless, their stories all converge in one simple, desperate question:

Why?

It's a question that comes in many variations:

- Why does this always happen to me?
- Why do I keep doing this to myself?
- Why am I always/never in this situation?
- Why doesn't that ever work out for me?
- Why don't things ever seem to go my way?
- Why can't I get what I want?
- Why is life so stressful?
- Why do I struggle so much?

- Why do I keep sabotaging myself?
- Why can't I achieve the success I want?

Some people would say that there is no answer to the "why" question—that life is just hard work, and that bad things happen to good people for no discernible reason.

I'm here to tell you that those people are dead wrong.

THERE IS AN ANSWER

Every effect has a cause. If you can get deep enough into the truth about suffering, you can always see how it makes sense within the situation's context. This is true even of global issues like natural disasters and economic depressions, as well as political and cultural feuds that go on for hundreds of years. All of these systemic problems have a root cause that can be found if you have the ability and patience to do the necessary detective work.

But we're not here to talk about those problems. We're here to talk about YOU.

Why do YOU suffer?

If you're like a lot of my patients, you may have read that question and thought, "Wow, where do I begin?"

Let me help by listing a few possible reasons you might be suffering right now:

- You're constantly experiencing some level of stress.
- You're unable to have the kind of relationships you really want.
- Your health is getting worse and worse, despite your best efforts.
- Your family is divided and pulling you in different directions.
- Your child is caught in a harmful spiral.
- You're grinding away at a job where you never feel successful.
- You're locked in an emotional pattern that, no matter how clearly you see the harm it's causing, you just can't seem to quit.
- Despite managing your job, relationships, and health with success, you can't seem to muster up any joy in your life.

OKAY...BUT *WHY?*

From time to time, we all find ourselves experiencing the opposite outcomes from what we want. But why are you haunted by the same situations being repeated over and over again?

After all, you're a smart person. This isn't the first book you've read about how to fix your issues and live your best life. So why are those issues still controlling you? Why haven't you been able to be the best person you can be?

I'll tell you why: it's because you don't even know who that person is.

LIVING IN INTEGRITY

Most people grow up completely ignoring themselves without even realizing it. They form a concept of Self based on all kinds of false expectations, without ever making a conscious connection to the true Self they were born to become. Over time, this true Self keeps trying to make itself known. But because conventional "maturity" usually consists of learning new and clever ways to mask or ignore the true Self, we continue to stifle it, pacify it, and drown it out.

Is it any wonder that so many people go through life feeling lost? Instead of living their true lives, people are living false narratives. Or, as I call it, "living out of integrity." The result is stress, pain, suffering, confusion, and chaos. Every joy is watered down, every epiphany is muted, and every triumph loses its shine, because it has little or no connection with its authentic purpose and potential. When a person lives out of integrity with their true Self, the best they can hope for is survival.

What's more, every therapeutic approach fails miserably because—get this—it's being applied to a Self that isn't *you*.

I realized this truth after years of helping people as a friend and colleague, but years before I became a clinical psychologist. I loved helping people, and I took it upon myself to delve deeply into every avenue—from science to spirituality to nutrition—to give people the resources they needed to transform their lives.

From the beginning, I could see that all patterns of suffering were related to this same issue of being out of integrity with the true Self. This was underscored by certain people I'd encounter who were so profoundly disconnected from themselves that no matter how successfully they managed life, they could not feel fulfilled or happy. For these people, no insight or technique I could offer would help, because the person was applying them to a mistaken identity; it would have been like taking someone else's medication and expecting their own illness to be healed.

That's when I realized it was time for a whole new approach to my work. I couldn't truly help people until I revealed what I'd discovered long ago: all our maladies, neuroses, and Self-destructive patterns are connected at the core. Once I could see how a single core issue exacerbates all the others, I could simplify the approach to fixing them and kill about a thousand birds (or more!) with one stone.

This is the approach that I now call The Method.

MEET THE METHOD

The Method is a way of being true—in thought, speech, and action—to the deepest essence of who you are. It helps you connect to the Self you *would* be if you were not afraid and habituated to believe that actually being your Self would somehow ruin your life. Far from being something dangerous, your true Self is your North Star. It has all the information necessary to guide you on the path to your purpose and potential.

Applying The Method uncovers your Self a little at a time. The more your Self is revealed, the easier it becomes to apply The Method. Even after using The Method for twenty years, I'm still amazed at how quickly my patients move forward on the path of their purpose and potential once they create this feedback loop.

If you've been to a lot of therapists over the years, I know this approach may sound too practical to you—maybe even ridiculously simple. But why shouldn't it be simple? Could it be that the only reason your life seems so hard, and so complicated, is because you expect it to be that way?

I live and work in a community of very effective, educated, and skilled therapists who work in every modality you can imagine. I regard most of them with boundless respect. But, if I'm honest, I can't believe that more of them haven't grasped the crucial truth that lies at the heart of our healing-obsessed culture: that health, fulfillment, and happiness come naturally when you allow life to be practical.

A lot of my colleagues look at me with one eyebrow raised when I say that my office is practically a revolving door. I don't keep patients for very long for the simple reason that, once they learn to cultivate a relationship with their true Self, they don't need help from me anymore.

And I wouldn't have it any other way.

That's why I wanted to write this book: to get this truth into more people's hands. Plus—I'll admit it—there's a bit of a selfish motive, too. After years of working with patients—people suffering from borderline personality and bipolar disorders, addiction, and eating disorders, along with plenty of your average Self-saboteurs—I have realized that my true Self is most fulfilled when I can introduce The Method to people who are desperate to discover the practical path to living their purpose and potential. The Method is so important because everyone has a deep desire to bring their gifts, talents, and innovative ideas to the world. My mission is to give America back its greatest asset: people who are living their purpose and potential. It kills me every time I have to turn away a patient because of my overbooked schedule, or cut a conversation short after a speaking gig, because I need to catch a plane. Putting The Method into this book is the next step forward on my own practical path.

So, for my sake as well as yours, I'm overjoyed that this book found its way into your hands.

FAIR WARNING

Having said that, I have to warn you of a few things:

1. THERE IS NO BULLSHIT IN THIS BOOK.

I get the need for empathy, understanding, and gentleness. But let's be honest—you've cried on enough therapists' couches. It's time to stop dwelling on the pain and start moving forward!

I'm writing this book the same way I conduct sessions in my office. We only spend enough time on your pain points to identify the starting place on your practical path. I know you may still feel fragile or vulnerable at this point, but I promise that your true Self is ready for this shift. You'll be so excited by the results that you won't miss the old "velvet glove" approach.

2. THERE ARE SOME NEW CONCEPTS YOU'LL HAVE TO GET USED TO.

The Method is based on living in integrity with your true Self. Learning to do this means accepting that the person you think you are is not the person you're truly meant to be. Prepare yourself for a good amount of forehead slapping and frequent rushes of blood to the brain. You're about to discover a whole new person living inside you. (Don't worry—I think you're going to really, really like that person.)

3. THINGS ARE GOING TO CHANGE.

You're going to be amazed at how easy The Method makes it to shift your life in the direction of your purpose and potential. For some people, it's a little bit *too* easy. The transition freaks them out. Most of us are so used to health and happiness being a slow, difficult process that the ease and practicality of The Method can take some by surprise.

Try not to be scared off by the *whoosh!* effect of putting The Method into practice. Again, once you experience the results of using The Method, these sudden shifts are exciting, enjoyable, and even a little bit addictive.

To ease you into this book, I'll start with walking you through the basics of The Method, showing you how it works and explaining the scientific and spiritual tenets that support it.

Next, I'll give you a deeper glimpse into how The Method was developed by walking you through the very first case study of how it worked...on me!

Then the rubber will hit the road—we'll take a deep dive into The Method together. I'll walk you through how to use The Method to create your practical path, day by day and moment by moment, at every level of your life.

YOUR TIME HAS FINALLY ARRIVED

They tell us life isn't easy.

They say that for some people, lasting transformation just isn't possible.

But maybe that's what they want us to think.

Maybe those people who are telling you how difficult it is to change are afraid of what you will become. Maybe they're afraid that if you connected to your purpose and potential, you'd allow them less control over your life. Maybe they're afraid if you break out of familiar patterns and refuse to live under the labels they've given you, it would disrupt their lives and make them really deal with truths of their own.

Let's give them a surprise, shall we? By working through The Method together, we'll show the world how amazing life can be when we live in integrity.

Pain and suffering have taken up enough of your time. Starting today, you get to officially dismiss them from the place they've occupied in your life. It's time for you to step onto your practical path—it's been waiting for you all along.

Before proceeding to chapter one, take a few moments to set yourself up for success by reviewing **Getting the Most Out of This Book**. The more you get out of this book, the more you'll experience your full potential each and every day of your life!

Chapter One

INTRODUCING THE METHOD: IT'S THAT EASY

———

You know that feeling you get when everything is going well in your life—you nailed that presentation, that special someone asked you out for a second date, your parents finally said they were proud of you—but somehow you still don't feel the deep glow of satisfaction that you expected to feel?

Friends may ask you what's wrong and you can't think of an answer. The best you can come up with is a vague admission, "Something's just missing."

When you think about it, that phrase is really powerful.

It speaks to the fragmented nature of most people's lives. Even when we have it all, there is still a part that doesn't feel complete.

"LIVING IN INTEGRITY" DEFINED

If you're like me, you've had those times in your life when it was abundantly clear that the pieces didn't fit together.

This confusion is at once totally normal and totally unprecedented. There's no good reason why we should be so confused about who we are, except for the fact that it's more normative for us to operate out of a misplaced, fragmented sense of Self. Our parents were raised that way, their parents were raised that way, most of our friends have been raised that way—why should we be any different?

But that's what you and I are here to change.

Think about the people you know who seem to live in a state of grounded bliss. They may be fabulously wealthy or just getting by. They may have a big, happy family, or they may live in solitude. It doesn't really matter, because something about them transcends all the circumstances in their lives. Whatever they're doing, they make it look easy.

These are people who are living in integrity. The pieces

of their lives are correctly identified, ordered, and fit into the correct whole. They know their purpose and are living their full potential every day, practically and naturally, in every situation.

This is the single thing people in pain truly need. Once the pieces of their lives are connected with their purpose and they can live their potential—no matter how much drama, disorder, or damage surrounds them—all their pain undergoes a dramatic reduction.

This is what makes The Method so incredibly effective. As I tell my clients over and over again when they can't believe the way their lives are finally beginning to take shape, "Yes, it's that easy!"

A WHOLE NEW YOU

We're connecting the pieces of your life with your purpose and potential in a way that seems like a whole new you. Except, it's the you that was there all along. It's just new to you because you've never met it before.

This shift is so monumental that it takes some people a few days to adjust. Having their true Self emerge is as startling as having their hair changed overnight from stick-straight to wildly curly. (If you're already rocking the curls, imagine it the other way around.) They may like their new (true) Self, but they don't quite understand how to work with it yet.

What guides you in living in integrity is your internal navigation system. Like your true Self, that system has been there all along. However, you've been taught to ignore it in favor of other people's expectations.

The Method will teach you to develop the practice of noticing and checking in with your internal navigation system. Once you begin to honor it, you'll find it signaling you more clearly. The more you listen to it, the more it will tell you, and the easier it will be for you to follow its guidance on your practical path, while kicking other people's expectations to the curb.

But it gets even better. By listening to your internal navigation system, you are creating a relationship with your Self. This is the most important relationship you will ever have. Learning to trust your internal navigation system is what makes it possible for you to live your purpose and potential. This is the mechanism behind The Method—the secret of its power.

A WORD OF ADVICE BEFORE WE START

Rebuilding the relationship with your Self is a lot like

building any relationship. It requires time, trust, and communication. Like a lot of the high-functioning people I work with, you may have developed these skills to a super-human degree in other relationships, but never put them to use on your Self. If so, you may regard the process I'm about to describe as being too precious, too Self-indulgent, too symptomatic of First World problems.

If that's what you're thinking, I have this to say to you:

Get over it.

You are not too cool for this. Your Self is begging you for a chance to really come through. Until you give it that chance, you're going to stay in pain. And guess what? It doesn't relieve anyone's pain, in the First World or anywhere else, for you to stay in pain.

Physical or emotional hurt is just the tip of the iceberg. The real toll of being in pain is the lost potential of living at your best in each moment. But now, by holding this book in your hands, you have an opportunity to leave the pain behind and begin living out your full purpose and potential. In doing so, not only will you benefit from all the skills, strength, and spiritual power your true Self has to offer, but you'll be benefiting the world around you at the highest possible level.

Ready to get to work?

Good. Let's get started.

INTRODUCING THE METHOD

One of my favorite aspects of The Method is how it marries the clinical with the spiritual. It pulls its three main elements from evidence born out of neuroscience and behavioral science, but also from intuitive and energetic practice. The result is a holistically practical path to finding your purpose and fulfilling your potential.

The Method rests on three main elements:

- Radical Self-inquiry
- Positive and assertive Self-talk
- Taking action on what you know to be true

These three elements can be applied either sequentially or simultaneously, depending on the situation. The main point is that they are all working for you from the moment you wake up until the moment you fall asleep.

Let's go through them one by one.

Nothing, and I mean nothing, happens to us without our telling ourselves a story about it.

Here are just a couple of examples of how we tell ourselves stories. One is pretty small, the other is big, but they revolve around the same central principle. As you read, see if you can figure out what that principle is.

EXAMPLE #1

You were really looking forward to spending the evening on your own, playing with your dog, maybe even working on a song you've been trying to write. But then, you get a text from a friend about a last-minute birthday celebration happening that night. You think, "I should go...I'm a bad friend if I don't celebrate my friend's birthday." An hour later, you're at the party trying to look like you're having a good time, until your friend says, "You know, if you're going to be in such a bad mood, you should have just stayed home."

EXAMPLE #2

You have a bad day at work and, as soon as you get in the door of your apartment, you've got the TV on and the wine bottle uncorked. Hour by hour passes as glass after glass goes down, while the same thought keeps running through your head, "This job is ruining my life, but I can't leave it—I have to keep a roof over my head."

Did you catch the uniting principle? What did both stories involve?

That's right—a choice about your behavior that was hidden under the belief that you *didn't* have a choice.

Telling ourselves stories is an instinctive way to process the world and identify ourselves within it. But because so much of what we tell ourselves is inaccurate, exaggerated, and missing important details, these stories end up amounting to outright lies. These lies subconsciously reinforce our choices about acting in ways that seldom help us and usually cause us harm.

Neuroscientists have shown via functional magnetic resonance that the human brain operates as two systems. System #1, located within the basal ganglia, is where our brain processes primal instincts. It lights up when we smell delicious food, feel sexually aroused, or sense danger. System #2 is the rational part of our brain. Located in the neocortex, it lights up whenever we are having a conversation, reading a book, or thinking conscious thoughts.

Now, which system do you think is responsible for the

majority of our choices? Would it surprise you to learn that 90 percent of our decisions are made by System #1? Neuroscientists report that while System #1 is directing our path, System #2 is usually relegated to creating a rationalization—a "story"—to support whatever urges System #1 might have at any given time.

However, System #2 does in fact have the ability to override our primal instincts with logic and rational thought. But it can only do this if we hold ourselves to strict accuracy with the stories we tell ourselves. This is where radical Self-inquiry comes in.

Next time you tell yourself a story, take a few minutes to review it. Did that story make you feel good? Did it highlight your value as a person? Did it help you achieve more of what you wanted or how you wanted to feel?

Or, did that story cause you pain? Did it emphasize your weakness? Did it provoke grief, hatred, despair, or resentment?

Finally, what did that story make you want to do next? Was it to "go out and conquer the world," or was it more like "crawl into a hole or take a baseball bat to someone's windshield?" Did the story motivate you to make the most of each moment, or did it sidetrack you into a fantasyland?

It's important to notice these things without judgment of yourself or others involved in the story. Judgment only serves to create a new story to sort through. Stick with the one at hand and ask yourself the final question about this story, "Is it true?"

Let's pick apart the examples I gave a moment ago.

EXAMPLE #1

- Before this party invitation came along, would you have described your Self as a bad friend to this person?
- In this particular case, why *should* you do something that you really don't want to do? Why *should* you choose someone else's plans over the ones you made for the evening?
- Would you be acting in integrity with your Self by going to the party? Would you be in integrity with your friend by attending their party when you really don't want to be there?

EXAMPLE #2

- Is your current job really the only way to keep a roof over your head?
- Is your dissatisfaction with your job the consistent source of bad symptoms, like that bottle of wine you've nearly finished?
- Is it the job that's the problem, or is it the career? In

other words, do you love what you do but not where you're doing it?

- Are there ways that you could improve your work life? If so, what's keeping you from taking those steps?
- What were the reasons that led you into that career in the first place? Are those the reasons you want to use to make your choices in the future?

As you might imagine, System #2 in your brain will supply plenty of quick reasons to stay locked in the habitual crisis mode of System #1. You'll find your Self knee-deep in something called "confabulation." This term has become a lot better known in recent years, thanks to psychologist Brené Brown introducing it on Oprah's "Super Soul Sunday." It refers to telling your Self lies that you honestly believe to be true. This belief may come from taking someone else's word for it, incorrectly interpreting the feedback you get from the world around you, or simply buying into a cliché that is so familiar you've forgotten to question it anymore.

But these confabulated stories are like amateur poker players—they have tells. One big one is the phrase, "I should." If you find yourself thinking, *I should/I have to/I've got to/I need to*, it's a good indication that an untruth is about to come out.

Here's another example to go along with the birthday

party scenario above: "I've got to finish this paperwork before I go home tonight."

Is that statement 100 percent true?

Is it true that you would lose your job tomorrow if you didn't complete this task tonight?

Or, would it be more accurate to say you dislike waking up to a lot of paperwork? If that's the case, you're empowered to make a decision between two preferences—going home now and accepting that you'll have some paperwork tomorrow, or finishing your paperwork first and going home later. Whatever you choose to do, *you're* the one in charge, not some needless "I have to" stress related to a confabulated story you've told your Self.

Another *tell* of the false narrative is the physical or emotional response that follows from it. False narratives not only provoke actions that are out of integrity with your Self, but they also have a habit of provoking reactions. False stories create a pattern of stressful dysfunction in your life, which in turn creates physical dysfunction in the form of chronic illness. If you routinely come down with a migraine or get unusually irritable or tired after a certain situation, it's a sign that you've been living within a false story about that situation.

Some false stories are harder to disown than others. You may have doubts about whether a given story is true or not. It's okay if this happens. The key here is to rigorously stop telling yourself things that you don't *absolutely know* are true. It's better to silence your inner voice and leave that space open for a while. Eventually, the truth will begin to make itself known to you.

In Chapter 7, we'll talk about how to catch these false stories in real time. For now, know that the more you practice this radical Self-inquiry, the more easily you'll adapt to the second element in The Method.

ELEMENT 2: POSITIVE AND ASSERTIVE SELF-TALK

Your brain can be very loud and assertive with its false stories. Therefore, positive change demands that you be equally loud and assertive with your positive speech.

By positive, I don't mean irrational optimism. Instead, I use "positive" to mean the assertive form of speech that is productive, supportive, affirming of what *is* instead of what *isn't*.

I warn you, this will feel awkward at first, since every cell in your body may have been operating according to a false story for years. Don't be surprised if you feel like a fraud the first few times you correct your false narrative with the truth. The more you practice this rigorous truth-telling, the more your brain will begin to reinforce it for you. That's just how brains work. They're shockingly easy to persuade.

Successful use of The Method demands that you be 100 percent accurate in what you tell your Self. No speculating allowed. If you don't *absolutely* know something to be the truth, don't say it. Don't give yourself permission to be a liar about your life. Instead, have fun exploring the truth inside you.

Let's apply this to the examples above. Here is what you might say to your Self once you've recognized the false narratives:

EXAMPLE #1

"There's no reason I *should* go to this party. I'm a good friend to So-and-So—I don't need to prove it by going out tonight. Even if she's mad at me for not being there, our history is deep enough that skipping this party tonight won't ruin our friendship. I trust that my love for her is stronger than my fear of not being loved by her."

EXAMPLE #2

"It would be good to keep a roof over my head because I care about my Self. But I am a free individual—there is literally nothing in this world that I *have* to do. I see that I want a different kind of experience in my career, something that enhances fulfillment in my life. I also enjoy the experience of having a nice home to live in. I have the power to create what I want, and I acknowledge that I'd like to evolve my life so that I have both a nice home and a career that I love. I am going to focus on the truth of what I really want and the creative ways that I can work towards having more of what I want overall in my life. It may take some effort and creativity, but I am committed to my Self in finding the path to fulfillment."

Let's throw a third example into the mix, one that's a true therapy classic:

"I want to get along with my father, but it probably isn't possible. He doesn't love me as much as I love him."

While I agree that lack of love is a possibility in any parent-child relationship, it's a lot less common than many children believe. So, I'll typically challenge this assertion with my clients by asking whether they really know that to be true.

"Has your father told you he doesn't love you?" I'll ask. "Has he never once showed evidence of loving you, such as providing food and shelter, taking you somewhere special, bringing you a gift, calling you on the phone?"

Parents can be incredibly bad at showing love, but it doesn't mean the love isn't there. So, if you can't offer watertight, conclusive proof of your father not loving you, then that story is, as they say in court, inadmissible. Repeating this narrative will only drive continuous pain, loss, grief, hopelessness, and powerlessness in your relationships.

So instead, let's explore the positive truths around your feelings—the things you can be 100 percent sure of. You can say with perfect certainty that you love your father and that you want to feel more connected to him than you currently do.

Keeping your Self-talk to 100 percent verifiable accuracy usually means exchanging negative, destructive, insulting inner narration for positive, assertive statements. Your positive Self-talk may be tentative at first, full of caveats and apologies to an imaginary crowd. But eventually that Self-consciousness will fall away, and you'll soon be affirming your Self without hesitation, apology, or excuses.

What's more, once you begin communicating with your

Self this way, you will find your Self naturally communicating with others in the same way. You have no idea how powerful this kind of communication—unapologetic, unhesitant, affirmative, and direct—can be until you try it. (We'll get more into this in Chapter 9.)

Let's take a very trivial example: you need to push back a 9 o'clock appointment with someone. Rather than texting them and saying, "I'm running late, so sorry, here's what's going on..." you send a simple, direct, positive message, "I'll be there at 9:12."

Believe it or not, you've done a lot in these few words. Aside from sparing someone a boring and belabored apology, you haven't supplied them with reasons to be upset with you. That means that when you do show up, the meeting won't start off on a negative foot. You've also given that person the ability to take their time; now they don't have to rush. Because let's be honest—they're probably running late, just like you.

Saying "I'm late" is a judgment on yourself in the situation. The purpose of this judgment is to protect yourself from the other person's displeasure. "They won't judge me if I judge myself first," goes the rationale. But think about it. Why offer the other person a judgment of your Self, when you have no idea if they would have judged you anyway?

Saying, "I'll be there at 9:12" makes the situation neutral, allowing the other person to do their own thinking. If they need to advocate for themselves in the situation, give them the space to do so. But you'd be surprised how insignificant these things are to other people, when we don't make them a big deal with our overproduced apologies.

While it's important to acknowledge another person's feelings about how your actions have affected them, trusting your internal navigation system means believing that even when your actions have unintended consequences, you are still on the right path. Rather than letting those consequences bog you down, you offer the necessary communication and keep moving forward. Every action you take, regardless of the consequences, is part of the process of uncovering your true Self and giving it a chance to shine.

YOUR INTERNAL NAVIGATION SYSTEM

By now you may be wondering just who is this true Self we keep talking about? And how do I know when I've found it?

Easy. Your internal navigation system will tell you.

The internal navigation system is the signaling mechanism that is always trying to direct you back to your purpose and potential. Your internal navigation system is built on the unique, unrepeatable foundation of your true Self. You were born with it, and it has always been and will always be inside you, giving you clear, practical guidance on the path you were meant to live.

However, nearly everyone is conditioned to distrust their internal navigation system. As a result, they go off course from their practical path. I did this for much of my life; you've been doing it for much of yours. It's okay—it's easy enough to get back on your path. You just have to start following the guidance of your internal navigation system.

Finding your Self is not as big a mystery as people make it out to be. Your internal navigation system has been at work inside you since you were a child, guiding you to pick one toy instead of another. Your Self always knows when you are out of integrity by believing a story that is untrue. Your Self knows when you are putting that story into action, reinforcing its power over you. Your Self knows that the real source of the pain that you battle each day is the result of being disconnected with your purpose and potential.

That pain is the first place to start as you learn how to listen to your internal navigation system. Pain, stress, and discomfort are distress signals from your internal navigation system in response to living out of integrity with the purpose and potential of your true Self. This pain might be physical, such as chronic migraines, digestive issues, or a life-threatening disease. It might also manifest as crippling anxiety, depression, or mental illness.

This pain should, in some ways, be reassuring. Your internal navigation system will never let you stray from your path without a fight. We'll go into more detail about the "tuning in" process in the next chapter; for now, I'll just say it's a lot less mysterious or difficult than you might expect. If you can just allow your Self to notice when and where these pain signals happen, you can begin to shift your attention from the false story you've been acting out to the true story that is begging to take its place.

ELEMENT 3: TAKING ACTION ON WHAT YOU KNOW TO BE TRUE

Self-realization doesn't end with epiphany or mental consent. It requires you to take action. Not only does action express your true Self in a given moment, but it also sets up a new feedback loop to reinforce the bigger concept of living in integrity. Each time you act in integrity, you send signals to your entire mind-body-spirit complex: "This is what we're doing now." Before long, your entire Self-concept begins to change.

The final step in The Method is taking action on the true

stories. And guess what? Stories that are 100 percent true lead you to actions that are 100 percent doable for you!

Let's go back to our previous examples.

EXAMPLE #1
You text your friend back and say, "Happy birthday! Thank you so much for inviting me, but I already made plans for tonight. I look forward to setting up a time to get together when we are both available so we can celebrate and catch up. Have a great time!"

EXAMPLE #2
You reflect that a big change, like a career shift or finding a new job, is not an overnight fix. You acknowledge that the first and most important step you can take in this moment is being non-judgmentally honest about whether a wine and TV binge is getting you closer to the life you want, or if it's taking you further away.

In the case of connecting with your father, there are so many options for how you can live the true story of how you feel toward him! You can call your father, you can visit him, you can send him a gift or a note that expresses your love, or you can simply crack open a photo album to revisit the good times you've had with him.

To facilitate building this feedback loop, you need to follow each act of integrity by checking in with your Self. Pay attention to what happens when you act in integrity, compared to what used to happen when you didn't. For example, if you used to get migraines or experienced digestive discomfort every time you made a choice that was out of integrity with your Self, what kinds of feelings do you get when you act in integrity? Some people get a little lightheaded, while others feel a burst of energy or creativity, or experience a rush of love and positivity.

Sometimes, the check-in may even reveal a deeper layer of your true Self. It may uncover a Self-defeating attitude, belief or action that you never realized was there. This will be proof that The Method is working. It's digging deeper into the layers of untruth built up by parenting, schooling, relationships, and the negative feedback loop that reinforced them all.

As we go deeper into this book, you'll learn more about how to act in integrity with your Self more consistently, and how that practice reaches the highest and most detailed levels of your life.

For now, though, you can begin taking the actions to change the situation. Certain changes may take a while—trust your Self and the work you're doing. Nothing changes if you don't put your discoveries into practice. Moving forward on your practical path means taking action on what you know to be true today so you can live your potential for the rest of your life.

.

Chapter Two

TUNING INTO THE INTERNAL NAVIGATION SYSTEM

One of the hardest things about living in the world today is distinguishing your true Self from all the other influences, voices, and thinking patterns that swirl within your psyche.

Is your Self the voice of panic screaming that your life is about to go up in flames?

Or is it that other voice telling you that you're freaking out just like your mom always did, that you'd better shape up or you're going to turn out just like her?

Or is it the person binge-watching TV in hopes of drowning out both of those voices?

Or is it the "ugh, not again" feeling that hovers over the whole mess?

Which one is your true Self?

I've got good news for you: none of them are.

Go ahead and breathe a sigh of relief.

YOU ARE THE SELF YOU HOPED YOU'D BE

Aren't you glad to learn that none of those voices were your true Self? Let's be real—none of them were very helpful, loving, or even nice to be around. If that's what your true Self was like, you'd have good reason for avoiding it all the time.

Fortunately, your Self is actually very lovable, interesting, smart, and insightful. There are no dark flaws, ugly awkwardnesses, or resident demons that you need to be afraid of. Instead, your Self is not only fully aware of its adorable idiosyncrasies, but finds them endlessly entertaining. Your Self enjoys being this interesting, unique person far more than following a one-size-fits-all social script.

This Self is not only someone you're sure to enjoy having a relationship with, but it's someone your family, friends, and coworkers would also really enjoy. But, before they get to know the real you, you have to cultivate a relationship with your Self that allows you to fully inhabit that Self.

In order to do that, you have to tune into your internal navigation system.

WHAT DOES "TUNING IN" MEAN?

It wasn't long ago that psychotherapists commonly equated the Self with an individual's thoughts. If a patient confessed to having crazy thoughts, they were diagnosed as being a crazy person. In the last several years, though, we've finally grown out of that belief, largely thanks to Eckhart Tolle and his seminal book, *The Power of Now*.

In his book, Tolle introduces the fundamental concept of the "observer," the part of an inner Self that transcends all our tangled, contradictory thoughts with an ability to hear and process without judgment. This nonjudgmental aspect is key to making a healthy choice about what to do with those thoughts.

Tolle's concept has empowered people tremendously to make distinctions amongst their emotions, the thoughts behind those emotions, and the behavior that stems from those emotions. By reassuring us that we are more than just the things we think, feel or do, this concept puts us back in the driver's seat of our own lives.

In some ways, Tolle's "observer" is just a reinterpretation of the familiar concept of intuition. In our information-glutted society, intuition empowers people to tune out the noise and return to the primal wisdom of "trusting your gut." The literal interpretation of this practice happens to be borne out by some amazing scientific research showing how the gut is flooded with stress-induced cortisol before the brain even recognizes the presence of a threat.

Whether you think of intuition as a signal from your intestinal bacteria or from something more ephemeral, the point is that something inside you knows what is good for you before you even have to think about it.

A third teaching you may be familiar with is the Buddhist practice of mindfulness. This practice asks you to enter a state of quiet coexistence with your thoughts. You let them enter and exit at will, acknowledging them without being provoked or perturbed. You're not above them, you're not below them—you're simply present with them.

All three of these concepts emphasize the truth that you

are not your thoughts. No matter how insistent your internal monologue might be, there is something in you that can detach from your thoughts, find the core truth that they contain, and choose how that truth relates to your purpose and potential.

I'm a big fan of all these approaches to separating your thoughts from your understanding of Self. But with all due respect to Tolle and tradition, I find that they ultimately fall short when it comes to creating a practical path for living your life.

After all, the best these approaches can offer you is a reprieve from the craziness. What's more, they cultivate this notion that in order to make healthy, rational choices, you have to effectively step outside your Self and perform a therapy session on your own brain. And let's face it—in the midst of a crazy day at work or a heated conflict with your spouse, it's rare that you can call a timeout to stop, observe, get your Self grounded, and sit in calm presence. Even if you could, the craziness would still be waiting when you returned to the situation.

This is precisely why so many people give up on practices like meditation. It tells them to detach from regular life at a level that most of us cannot afford or just don't have the personality for. As a highly energetic person who thrives on living in flow, I have to tell you that traditional meditation—silent, still contemplation—is not a sustainable practice for me. As I told a client once, my life is my meditation. My clarity comes through kinetic connection with my purpose, which helps me live my full potential each day.

What makes The Method so different from more traditional intuitive approaches is that it identifies your internal navigation system in everything. Far from asking you to step outside your Self, The Method asks you to lean deeper into your Self by tuning into your internal navigation system right in the moment of conflict or stress.

The Method says that your internal navigation system is just as present within your crazy thoughts as it is within your cerebral "observer" and your gut-level intuition. Your internal navigation system is available to you whether you're feeling energetic or exhausted, high on life, or in the depths of despair. It's beside you when you uncork the bottle, get on the treadmill, pop the pills, send the text message...any time you say "yes" when everything inside you is screaming, "*No!*" In any situation, your internal navigation can tell you what's really happening, lead you back to your Self, and help you move forward in integrity on your path.

NON-JUDGMENT IS EVERYTHING

If there's one thing we all hate, it's hearing judgment in the voice of a family member or friend, especially when that judgment is hovering behind words like, "I say this because I love you," or "I just want the best for you."

But forget about judgment from others for a minute. When was the last time you really spoke to yourself without judgment? And I'm not just talking about feelings of guilt when you order dessert. I'm talking about the judgments you make that are disguised as humility, empathy, or even love.

For example, you give a great presentation and while everyone is offering their kudos, your brain whispers, "Finally, you did something that didn't completely suck."

As another example, you get off the phone with your dad after a pretty decent conversation, and your first feeling is one of relief that maybe, just maybe, he really does love you.

You see, the problem isn't so much that other people are judging you. It's that you have accepted judgment as a natural way to relate to someone, and you incorporate it into your relationship with your Self.

This is another way that traditional thought management

approaches can often fail people. Over time, this habit of judgment makes its way into your innermost psyche—it becomes *intuitive*. As a result, even your attempts to detach from your Self end up working against you. You're sitting there trying to meditate, but every time your Self tries to communicate to you, you feel like a failure because something "interrupted" your meditation.

When you eventually give up the practice—as so many people do, because nobody likes to keep doing something that makes them feel like a failure—you think, "Well, I'm a lost cause. I can't do the practice necessary to still my mind, so it looks like these destructive thoughts are just going to be here forever."

By contrast, The Method offers you the chance to believe the best about your Self no matter how far down the path of lies you find it. That's because your Self is constantly being guided by your internal navigation system. By tuning into it, you get to dispense with all judgment and use each situation to receive crucial information that will let you make the best and most practical choice for living your purpose and potential.

GIVE YOUR SELF THE ATTENTION YOU NEED

We've all seen what happens when a child is being ignored

by their parent or teacher. They start to repeat the same word over and over, hoping they will eventually be heard. Then they start to yell, stomp their feet, pound their fists. If the child continues to be ignored over a period of months or years, they start acting out in ways that are harmful to themselves or others.

This is essentially what your Self has been doing all your life. It desperately wants to be seen, heard, recognized, acknowledged, and allowed to express your purpose and potential.

Just like a neglected child, your Self is greedy for attention. But not for the attention of your father, your girlfriend, your boss, or even the world of social media. The only attention that will satisfy your Self—that will calm it down, soothe its frustration, and help it cease its negative behaviors—is attention from *you*.

Of course, most of us have been trained to believe that "attention seeking" is wrong. Maybe you've grown up hearing this message from parents, "Ignore her, she just wants attention." Maybe you've been accused by friends of always needing to be the center of attention when you go out. Maybe your partner has complained that you seem upset any time they pay attention to something besides you.

If that's the case, let me assure you that the only reason you've developed those exhibitionist behaviors or needy tendencies is because your Self was neglected and wanted attention...from *you*. Essentially, it was using your family and friends to alert you to the fact that there is a problem inside you. They can only see the signal flag your Self is waving—chronic stomachaches, compulsive shopping, oversensitivity, promiscuity. It's up to you to notice and address the real issues that are keeping your true Self from manifesting.

This is where the path to fulfilling your purpose and potential shows up: the moments where, instead of demanding that others recognize your needs, you choose to turn inward for the information that only your Self can provide.

LIVING IN INTEGRITY, DEMYSTIFIED

If you're like a lot of people, you have this vague idea that your true Self lies deep within you, inert under a lot of emotional baggage, bad teaching, and negative thinking patterns.

Maybe you've been told to tap into your intuition and let your Self be guided without thought.

Maybe you've tried to rationally observe and talk your Self down from the ledge of insanity.

Maybe you've dabbled with meditation in an attempt to still the mind and let the answer rise from within.

If these practices work for you, great. But the truth is that sometimes silence is just that: silence. It might be calming, but it doesn't actually tell you anything. It doesn't give you the direction you're craving. It doesn't respond to your fears with facts. It doesn't tell you anything relevant to the situation that is making you anxious, or giving you a migraine, or tempting you to drink, overeat, swallow the pill, send the text, or answer the call.

Unless you're planning to take up residence in a Zen monastery or live in a state of cerebral detachment, life pretty much demands that you do more than sift through your thoughts for clues as to which ones are valid expressions of your true Self.

Tuning into your internal navigation system is so much simpler than that. It doesn't make you wait for an answer about who you are; it assumes the answer is already there. By tuning into your internal navigation system, you can bypass the long sessions of Self-analysis or even silence. You can learn quickly to recognize the triggers that cause you stress and provoke destructive behavior.

As a result, the stress you experience starts to ease up.

Once your Self knows that you're paying attention to its signals, it doesn't have to make those signals so often or as intense. As the stomachaches become less severe, the blind rages die down, and the urge to compulsively shop, drink, or screw starts to evaporate, you find your Self contemplating the real feelings underneath those reactions—anxiety, sadness, envy, frustration.

This is where a lot of therapy stops—understanding the feeling, observing it, managing it. But what the internal navigation system will do is quite revolutionary—it will show you how to make the feeling go away.

Not just make you forget about it, like your behaviors did.

Not just observe it or analyze it to death or walk away from it.

Instead, your internal navigation system will help you take concrete, authentic action. Action that turns those negative feelings into joy, excitement, satisfaction, and gratitude. Action that leads you toward living in integrity with your Self. Action that puts you back on the path of your fullest potential in every moment of every day.

Remember how I said that information received without judgment will let you make the best choice for your Self? A lifetime of making those best choices is what I call living in integrity. Integrity cannot coexist with judgment, for the simple reason that judgment is divisive. By contrast, your internal navigation system is all about healing through reconciliation. Whatever information it receives, your internal navigation will insist on connecting that information in a positive way with your purpose and potential.

This starts with the information your mind and body send to your internal navigation, but it also works outward to the information your internal navigation absorbs about the world. None of us can live in a bubble, and your internal navigation will have to process its fair share of negative input. Accidents happen, circumstances change, and we all grow old.

But by living in integrity with your Self, you can acknowledge your losses without losing the potential in each moment. The internal navigation system will show you how to deal with disappointment, failure, and even tragedy in a way that increases your inner strength, spurs your growth, and lets your Self emerge triumphant.

LEARNING TO BE SELF-FUL

Long before you knew how to be mindful or access your intuition, you had this internal navigation system. It was there from the beginning of your life, and it was designed to make following your path practical, natural, and automatic. When you learned to walk, it told you when to walk toward your mother, and when to walk past her and go for the toy lying in the corner. When you got to preschool, it told you what color crayons to use and how much to eat at snack time. When you got to elementary school, it told you to be friends with a certain person, despite knowing nothing about them yet.

Over time, though, you began to apply a matrix of evaluation to the guidance given by your internal navigation system. This evaluation wasn't based on your ingrained connection to your Self (you didn't even know there was such a thing); instead, it was based on what you knew about the Self you believed you were supposed to be. You started being Self-conscious. You started second-guessing everything. You started judging your actions, preferences, desires, thoughts...again, not about whether they connected with your purpose and potential, but whether they matched with the person you thought you were supposed to be. This is the foundation for losing your potential—because you're losing the Self you were supposed to effortlessly be, which is, of course, your purpose. See how practical that is?

That judgment system may have been introduced by your

observation of others around you—parents, classmates, neighbors, friends. But it could just as easily have come from your own lack of knowledge about what to do with your thoughts and feelings. Since you never had the benefit of being taught about your internal navigation system as a child when the heavy introspection and conflicting emotions of adolescence set in, you didn't know what to do with it all. You probably looked around for people who seemed to be sure of themselves and observed that the people who were popular, athletic, and beautiful never seemed to suffer from embarrassment or insecurity. That's when you concluded that being more like that person meant being happier, more confident, and more successful at life. It probably never occurred to you that it might be the other way around—that being happy and confident with themselves could be what made them beautiful and popular.

Of course, you have no idea what that person's relationship to their Self was like. They could easily have been just as insecure as you were, but were better at playing the role of a false Self that they learned from someone else. It's also entirely possible they were 100 percent authentic, and their confidence was based on living fully in tune with their internal navigation system.

Either way, your attempt to solve your own Self-doubt by

modeling your Self after them only made your situation worse. Instead of tuning into your own internal navigation system, you set a precedent for living according to a false narrative of who you are "supposed" to be. That paradigm was likely encouraged by the example of other friends, not to mention parents and teachers. As author and teacher, Geneen Roth, sharply observes, "Often, the people who gave us these instructions are the sort we wouldn't ask street directions from today."

As a result of this false narrative, the person whom you now present to the world is completely hollow. It's just a prop, a shell. Your true Self doesn't live inside it.

If you've ever wondered why so many people feel so incredibly empty, this is the reason. We run ourselves ragged trying to keep busy, we throw ourselves at people who are too disconnected from themselves to take care of us, we bury ourselves in food, alcohol, or pills—all in an attempt to make ourselves feel full and complete.

But it doesn't work—it *can't* work—because these things are being consumed by a false Self, incomplete and disconnected. Meanwhile, the real Self—the one inside of you—is left feeling lonely, lost, and starving for attention.

Forget about mindfulness. What you really need is to start

practicing "Self-fulness"—intently focusing on feeding the true Self inside of you through following the guidance of your internal navigation system. Once you establish this connection to your true Self, then that desperate hunger you feel will immediately start to change. Your craving for unwholesome foods, your urge for toxic substances, your attraction toward destructive people...all of that will begin to shift in a palpable, real-time way. You'll be astonished at how differently the world looks once your internal navigation system starts calling the shots.

Best of all, your sense of moderation will kick in. You'll begin to feel when you've had enough—enough food, enough alcohol, enough entertainment, enough company. This happens because you'll no longer be worried about running out. You'll stop fearing that this will be the last time you'll experience love, pleasure, success, or freedom. Know why? Because you'll have begun to trust your internal navigation system to guide you to the things you need whenever you need them.

Does it take some practice to get to that point? Absolutely. Tuning in to your internal navigation system later in life is a lot like getting behind the wheel of a car after spending years riding the New York City subway. Your body vaguely recognizes the motions of driving, but your brain is second-guessing everything you do as you do it.

That's why you begin with checking in on small issues and work out toward ever-wider, ever-deeper levels. We'll get more into this process in Chapter 7. For now, just know that in the beginning, the process is fairly pedantic. You'll have to schedule brief check-ins with yourself to consult your internal navigation system about what it's telling you through various pains, emotions, and other triggers. These are the concrete actions that move you forward on your practical path. By building a caring, kindly curiosity about the real person that lies inside you, you're allowing your true Self to blossom.

After just a week of these regular check-ins, you'll find your brain's feedback loop taking over. You won't need to have these deliberate conversations with your internal navigation system quite as often. Instead, the communication between your inner whole Self and your outer fragmented behavior will start to happen on its own. As soon as you feel an external irritation, your internal navigation system will immediately and subconsciously guide you to respond with the actions, words, and even thoughts that connect to your truth, which is the experience of living your potential.

It's like a beautiful dance—the more time you spend with your partner, the more you trust them to make the moves that signal you to do your part. As this relationship with your Self grows, you can move more freely, express yourself more openly, and take risks more courageously.

SO WHAT HAPPENS NOW?

You might be wondering what happens once this process becomes seamless. When you give your internal navigation system free reign to guide you through the world, when you've developed a committed interest in your true Self, when you keep your Self filled with everything it needs to thrive...what does life look like then?

To start with, you'll find your life brimming over with a sense of purpose and potential. The healthy, nonjudgmental interest you've cultivated in your Self will naturally begin to extend toward other people. The attention-seeking behaviors that make other people pull away from you will start to dissipate. Instead, you'll become the person who is deeply interested in others, who is eager to listen, asks great questions, and sees the best in the people they meet. Don't be surprised if you find people saying they are drawn to you, complimenting and affirming you, and not only seeing but validating you for the amazing person that you are.

Think of a fountain, where the water only spills over once the pool is full. That is what your inner Self will be like.

You will be anchored by your sense of completeness. You will be sensitive to how much you have to give, and to when it's time to pull back and refill before you give out any more. Your internal navigation system will let you seamlessly recognize the people who appreciate you for who you are, and give you the ability to compassionately withdraw from the people who want something you cannot offer. You will be fully present in your life without fear. You will trust yourself, and you will not be wrong. You will experience, perhaps for the first time ever, what it feels like to be at peace.

Chapter Three

TELLING MY STORY...AND WHY IT MATTERS

———

What would you guess is the number one thing that prevents people in pain from seeking help?

It's not that they don't know help is available.

It's not even that they don't see how much they need it.

What stands in their way is that they don't believe that they deserve help.

For most of my adult life, despite all the work I put into healing myself mentally and emotionally, it never occurred to me that my challenges were the result of trauma in my childhood and teen years. Yes, I saw that I had issues. Yes, I acknowledged that I was unhappy. But trauma? That was a word for people who had suffered real tragedy. Not for me.

I came from a financially stable, upwardly mobile family. I knew that my parents and relatives loved me. I received a great education, enjoyed a lot of material blessings, had an amazing career, and built tremendous friendships that have lasted to this day.

What I didn't realize then (and has become so glaringly obvious to me now) was how many of us dismiss our painful experiences as being minor, trivial, and not worthy of being called "trauma." It might surprise you, but this is true across the spectrum of suffering. Even people who have been abused, abandoned, and marginalized for most of their life tend to downplay the trauma they have suffered.

We can all point to someone who had it worse than us. But what does that actually prove? It certainly doesn't help our own suffering go away. And it doesn't save us from perpetuating the legacy of trauma that we received onto the generations that follow us.

It makes me crazy when I hear suffering people (and sometimes even the therapists who treat them!) talk about healing as if it's a zero-sum game. Some of them seem to actually believe that the only way to grow as a person is through suffering—that if you've experienced or caused pain in your life, you must resign your Self to living with it from now on.

In my view, if you're in pain, you deserve to be told the pathway out of it—end of story.

The Method grew out of my personal realization that I deserved to heal from my pain. If you've lived in pain for a long time, you're acutely aware of how it prevents you from living your full potential and fulfilling your purpose. But what I finally realized was that not being connected to my true Self and living that in integrity was the opposite of my purpose. Living in that disconnection was stealing my potential every day, which further exacerbated the pain of not being my Self. Each moment I spent in pain held me back from using that moment to fulfill my purpose. Over time, those moments had created an entire life of missing my potential.

This was quickly followed by another realization: if nobody was going to take my pain seriously enough to help me, and if no one I knew seemed to be able to heal their own pain, then I would have to find healing on my own.

That Self-realization principle—that you can and must be the source of your own healing—is the foundation of The Method.

That's why I have no hesitation in sharing the specifics of my story with you, even if you and I come from completely different worlds. I've seen The Method transform people in every walk of life, from disenfranchised welfare dependents to über-rich scions of Silicon Valley, from ambitious but stifled artists to jaded white-collar professionals, to everyday trauma survivors being slowly zombified by medication. At bottom, we're all searching for the same thing: permission to connect with our Selves so we can live our life to its greatest potential, to become the person we know and secretly love, but whom we fear nobody will accept. Being ourselves is the only practical path through life. Any other way of life is confusing and chaotic, and in a constant state of performance, on the verge of breakdown, or being found out.

This is the imposter syndrome thing...it makes people feel like at any moment they will be discovered as a fraud or that everything will fall apart (breakdown).

Sometimes, though, it's easier to see this truth in someone else than in ourselves. So, let me share my story with you.

GROWING UP IN PAIN

Like so many children, I was a kid being raised by kids. My parents married way too young and by the time I came along, the pressures of adult life had significantly impacted their individual happiness and their relationship with each other. Life in their home was always an ordeal, fraught with tension and explosively volatile. It didn't matter whether the milk had spilled, or the car had been dented, or someone's feelings had been hurt—the sky was in a constant state of falling down.

My parents separated when I was six years old, which relieved the tension between them, but it didn't change their individual habits of dealing poorly with stress. Add in a slew of extended family members who also responded to life with high anxiety, oversensitivity, and loud voices, and you have an environment that, for a highly empathic child like me, translated into living in constant stress and pain.

You see how right off the bat, I can relate to people who feel the conflict of growing up in a safe and loving home but never feeling enough love and safety. Even though we always had food on the table and nobody was physically harming anyone, my childhood brain was being programmed like that of a kid living in a war zone. The fact is that for a growing child—even for a grown adult—

knowing that your family loves you is not the same as feeling truly loved.

Along with being a little sponge for other people's emotions, my personality was oriented to be a "fixer." This was the first and most foundational message I received from my internal navigation system: my purpose is to be a healer. You'll see as the chapter goes on how that purpose has directed my entire life and the experience of my potential. As a child, I simply couldn't run and hide under the bed or stare at the TV when the adults were fighting. Instead, I did my utmost to reduce the tension by being funny, entertaining, and caring. The last thing I wanted was to be yet another problem that made things worse for everyone.

MY FAMILY'S FIRST SHRINK

Strange as it may sound, the adults in my life began confiding in me as if I were a therapist. I can remember my uncle talking to me about my dad, my dad talking to me about my grandma, and my grandma talking to me about the rest of the family. She'd pick me up from school and we'd head to the bakery for a slice of cake, and as we sat there eating our dessert, she'd unload all the family situations she was worrying over: how this cousin was doing financially or why these two uncles weren't speaking to each other. By the time we'd finished our cake, she seemed to feel better.

I, on the other hand, felt paralyzed with thoughts and feelings that I couldn't express. I was too young to say what needed to be said: "Calm down and talk to each other like adults. You need to get past this pathological oversensitivity and start taking care of yourselves...and me! After all, I'm the child here." All I could do was pacify them by sitting there trying to absorb every frenzied emotion that was passed on to me.

To this day, I don't know if everyone thought I wasn't really listening or was just too young to understand all that they were saying. All I know is they kept burdening me with information that was wildly inappropriate for someone my age to hear—a burden that only grew heavier as I grew older. By the time I was twelve years old, I was lying awake at night thinking about these problems, while listening to the shouts of yet another family skirmish coming from down the hall.

COPING THROUGH FOOD

The message I was interpreting from my family was that life was incredibly hard, not just to live but to understand. I wondered if there was something wrong with me, since

I believed it shouldn't be this hard just to be alive. The question of who was the crazy one—them or me—generated serious anxiety in my young mind.

The burden of anxiety they gave me was one thing; the coping mechanism they gave me was another. Like so many women in western culture, the women on both sides of my family dealt with their feelings through food. Food denial, food indulgence, food fixation in thoughts, words, and actions. They were locked in a constant cycle of deny, binge, soothe, feel guilty, diet, repeat.

At the time when puberty arrived and body consciousness set in, my grandma began bringing me with her to Weight Watchers, as if it were an induction to womanhood. Those meetings taught me more about using food—both eating it and not eating it—to cope with the misery that seemed to be my birthright as a woman. By the time I reached age sixteen, disordered eating was just as regular a part of my life as homework after school and cartoons on Saturday mornings.

Oddly, despite all the strife in my family (or maybe because of it), we took great pride in coming off as well-adjusted, successful people. For my dad, that translated to a successful career, an ever-growing income, bigger houses, and BMWs. Following in his footsteps, I excelled in school while keeping a rigorous physical schedule for myself: up at 5:00 a.m. to run on the treadmill or ride the stationary bike, pushing myself in after-school sports practice, restricting calories throughout the day and then, just to be on the safe side, making myself throw up anything that I felt I hadn't "earned" through exercise.

Even if I could have articulated the emotional turmoil I felt, I wouldn't have known that the answer lay in loving my Self through the pain. The only model I knew for dealing with pain was to Self-medicate, primarily through food, and then to atone for that indulgence afterward. I had no concept that this "Band-Aid" approach only amounted to hurting myself still more.

My pain was compounded by my longing for my dad to see my problems and come to my rescue. I always had a suspicion that my dad wished I was a boy, that my being a girl made him uncomfortable. It seemed to me that once I began to transition from his cute little sidekick into a growing woman, he grew less and less interested in me. Empath that I was, I quickly intuited that my playing sports was something that gave him a lot of joy; so, instead of following my true extracurricular interests in theatre and music, I threw myself into basketball and track.

It just happened that I was a natural leader—the next

strong signal from my internal navigation system. In that regard, it didn't matter what activity I participated in—I was as dedicated to fostering team excellence in sports as I would have been in the arts. It also happened that my high school coach was a particularly great man who was more interested in his team's personal growth than in winning championships. He recognized that my athletic ability was far outshone by the strength of my personal drive to achieve excellence in whatever I did. So, when he coached me, it was all geared toward appealing to that inner drive. To this day, when I'm feeling uninspired or overwhelmed, his words still ring in my ear, "Don't give up, Thomas, you *got* this!"

My coach's message ultimately became a source of strength to do what I needed to do next: "come out" to my parents about my eating disorder.

THE LETTER AND WHAT CAME AFTER

The pain I felt was too great to hold inside anymore, but I still couldn't express it out loud. Instead, I wrote a letter to my parents describing how much I'd been suffering. I explained the pain I felt, described the Self-harmful ways I'd been dealing with it, and finished with a plea for them to find someone who could help me before it was too late.

I know it seems ludicrous that I had to actually write a letter to make my family notice my eating disorder. But isn't this typical of the way many of us grew up? Our family members are consumed with their own monumental issues; as children, we're just extensions of their own dysfunctional relationships to themselves, that they absorbed from their parents. They can't see us clearly because we're too close to them. My parents seemed so overwhelmed by their struggle with normal problems that their brains literally shielded them from seeing the life-or-death problem living within the body of their child. Even though they loved me more than anything in the world, they couldn't really see me.

My mom read the letter, shared it with my dad, and they took me to a psychiatrist. It only took a couple of sessions for the psychiatrist to see one of the major issues at play in my eating disorder: my deep desire for my dad to connect with me. He saw how badly I wanted to be acknowledged and loved for who I truly was, not as a sporty female substitute for a son.

I wish I could say that when the psychiatrist brought this up, my dad had a profound change of heart. But that's not how it went. Instead, he was outraged. Not only did he refuse to talk with the psychiatrist, but he even refused to pay for any more sessions.

You can imagine the lesson I took away from that: *Don't have pain, don't express pain, and definitely don't let Dad know you need his help with your pain.*

It took years before I saw what was really happening here. These people, my parents, didn't have the internal framework to recognize their own destructive patterns. They were entirely focused on building their lives, providing for their families, and getting ahead in life. Emotional needs were simply not on their radar. It's not surprising they were bewildered when their beloved child came to them openly for help. My dad didn't have the tools to accept his responsibility for the situation, and my mom was too overwhelmed to confront him about it or even find another outlet to get me help.

As a result, there was no result. We quit seeing the psychiatrist and life went on the way it had before.

LOOKING FOR LOVE...OR SOMETHING LIKE IT

The only option I felt I had left was to absorb back into myself the pain that my honesty had caused. At this point, sports became more of a refuge than ever. Every hour I spent playing basketball or running track was an hour where I could set aside the emotional baggage that weighed me down. It allowed me to concentrate on something simple, like rebounding the ball or leaping over the hurdle. And, of course, there was the uncomplicated, paternal presence of my coach, always laughing, always seeing my potential, and always encouraging me, "Don't be in your own head, Thomas; you *got* this!"

It was my coach who finally showed up with the rescue I'd been hoping for.

There was one springtime track practice where I was completely spent—wheezing, enervated, starving, exhausted. When all the other girls went to the showers, my coach had me take a seat in the grass and asked me quietly and without any drama, what was going on and what could he do to help.

It could have been my chance to get the help I needed, but I shied away from it. Instead, I told him I was upset over problems with my boyfriend.

This wasn't entirely a lie. My high school boyfriend was, like my eating disorder, just another symptom of my desperation for love and attention.

Clark was a sweet guy, very charismatic, full of admiration for how "together" I seemed, at least compared to him. A chronic low achiever, he was quickly following his own father's steps toward alcoholism. To him, I seemed like the smart, talented A-lister who had her life completely figured out. For my part, I loved seeing myself through his eyes. I also loved the way he made me feel pretty and desirable, instead of always having to be sporty and tough.

Of course, this was only how it felt when Clark was sober. When he was drunk, things changed drastically. He cheated on me; he yelled and called me names; he sometimes got physically violent. One time, when we were at a party, he got angry and pushed me right through a sliding glass door. The glass shattered and I fell to the ground, bruised, shaken, and humiliated. Everyone who saw it fully expected us to break up at that point (and probably hoped we would).

But we didn't. Even though I knew what we had was too toxic to be real love, I was addicted to the pedestal he put me on. By the time I graduated high school, I'd completely dismissed any belief that I was special, valuable, or deserving of admiration. In retrospect, I can see that having Clark admire me, being able to compare myself to him, let me feel like I was as special as I wanted to be. Though I didn't realize it at the time, I see now that something in me felt like being called a bitch or getting pushed around was a small price to pay for being recognized for the potential that I hadn't yet connected to.

Ever since, it has made perfect sense to me why people stay in bad relationships. When you feel as though your true Self has never been seen by those closest to you, it's hard to resist the allure of a relationship—even one that is unfulfilling, unhelpful, or downright toxic—with someone who does see you that way.

MISTAKEN MARRIAGE #1

The longer Clark and I stayed together, the more convinced I became that we would never work. Nevertheless, I didn't want to let the relationship go. Our dynamic, unhealthy as it was, felt familiar to me; after all, I'd been raised by people who quarreled, yelled, and treated themselves and each other poorly.

I was consumed with the effort to make our marriage work. At the same time, though, my internal navigation was desperately signaling me to get away before it was too late.

This was never clearer than the day when I said to Clark, "We've been together a long time. Aren't we going to get engaged?" Even as I said it, and Cinderella visions of dancing with my father at my wedding reception swirled around in my head, my internal navigation was telling me, "Tracy, you are a goddamn idiot."

I forged ahead with our wedding plans, knowing the whole time that it would be the stupidest thing I'd ever done. I knew this right up to the day my dad stood beside me at the back of the church. I looked down the aisle lined with our friends and family, saw Clark standing there beside the preacher, and thought these exact words, "I am 100 percent sure that I will not be with this person forever."

I know what it's like to look at the person you've been with for what seems like forever and think, "I can live with this." I know what it's like to believe that you can just strong-arm your way through the doubts and dissatisfaction, and that you'll get a fresh start once you take that next step in your relationship.

That's precisely what propelled me forward as I walked down that aisle, spoke my vows, and at age twenty-one, committed to living my life with a man I knew I shouldn't marry.

For about a year, Clark and I made it work, fighting constantly as I tried to make him become the healthy, happy person I wanted him to be for me. When I couldn't fix him, we both found refuge in our addictions—I Self-medicated with food, he with alcohol. Naturally, I did everything in my power to look as though I had it all together, just as I'd been trained to do. While I couldn't make my partner take care of himself, I could and did perform the hell out of my job, making ridiculous money for someone who was barely out of college.

For me, though, professional success wasn't all about the money. I was finding my natural place as a leader—someone who could tap into other people's psyches, help them connect to their potential in every task their role demanded, and motivate them to bring their best to their work. As a result, our team routinely shattered every revenue goal that was set for us, and I ascended the corporate ladder by leaps and bounds. In this one area of my life, I was really starting to tune into my internal navigation.

The next level of attunement came as a slap in the face. I mean a literal slap in the face. Clark and I were fighting and he hit me. I don't remember much else from that fight until his hands ended up around my throat. At that moment, it was like we both suddenly woke up. We were looking in each other's eyes, breathing raggedly, and knew without speaking that neither of us wanted to do this anymore. Not to each other, not to ourselves.

Again, I'd love to tell you that the weeks and months after that day were a series of revelations about listening to my internal navigation, understanding the role that I'd played in my own failed marriage, and consciously discovering the path to living my purpose and potential.

Instead, within a few years of divorcing, I was walking down the aisle toward a brand new man, thinking the same thoughts as I had the first go-round, "There's no way this is going to last."

MISTAKEN MARRIAGE #2

There's nothing like a divorce to whet your spirit's appetite for something new. I wanted to be around people who were powerful, intelligent, fabulous, and *knew* it. So, in 2001, I rented out my house in California, scored a new job and moved across the country to create my new destiny in Manhattan. I'd been dreaming of living there ever since watching *Sex and the City*, and the trajectory of my career had given me the confidence I needed to jump into big city life with both feet. Looking back, it was the first real decision made out of my internal navigation system, and the first step taken on my practical path.

Life in New York City was everything I expected and more. I was surrounded by people who were making things happen, were constantly striving for more, valued themselves highly, and demanded that others show them respect or get the hell out of the way. I found myself having intense conversations with some of the smartest people in the world, exulting in the city's cultural and social riches with some of the most interesting characters I'd ever encountered. I was marinating in a sea of movers and shakers, and learning from them how to connect with even more of my potential.

David and I got married in California, then moved together to Manhattan. He was nothing like Clark. He was kind, compassionate, and sweet, a gentleman to everyone, and an angel toward me. He made it easy to tell my Self the story that my first marriage had failed because I was a good girl married to a bad guy. I felt sure that things would be different now that I'd found a man who didn't have a mean bone in his body.

However, what David did have was $50,000 worth of debt. If I'd been listening to my internal navigation, I would have seen this for what it was: a symptom of a much deeper issue with how he treated himself. But once again, I jumped into a relationship as the healer, ready to take on another romantic partner as my "client."

Looking back, I can't fully blame myself for making these terrible choices regarding my life partner. It was just an underestimation of my own worth, combined with a misinterpretation of my purpose and potential. I wasn't living in my truth, and I experienced less potential than I should have. My navigation was guiding me toward a deep, soul-level connection; I just didn't realize that it was supposed to be with my Self.

Moreover, I was definitely more confident helping someone else reach their highest capacity than acknowledging my own. I saw the good parts of these men and felt that my own well-being depended on staying connected to them and helping them become better versions of themselves, rather than seeing how their weaknesses could hold me back. I had been taught to think that going through another person was how I reached my potential.

If you change out the fights for long, sad silences, my second marriage was almost beat for beat the same as the first—buy a new house, succeed at work, fail at fixing my partner and finally, three years later, file for divorce.

It broke my heart to break David's heart, and the guilt and pain might have driven me over the edge—or worse, into yet another terrible marriage—if it hadn't been for one thing: *The Oprah Winfrey Show*.

SELF-HELP

Ever since I was fifteen years old, I'd been following

Oprah's career. My grandmother and I transitioned from cake and ice cream dates to tuning in to our local ABC affiliate to watch Oprah talk to extraordinary people about overcoming everyday problems. Week by week, she was introducing me to the idea that there was a "best Self" somewhere inside me, and that making contact with it would help me feel okay in my own skin. In some ways, it was the gradual infiltration of this idea that prompted me to write my letter to my parents, to confess the truth to my coach, to have me relocate my life to Manhattan, and to acknowledge my leadership potential that was guiding my career to greater heights of success.

It was because of Oprah's teaching and her encouragement to journal that I moved to New York. It also helped me initiate the second divorce, despite the sadness I felt about it. During that time, guided largely by Oprah's recommendations, I dove deeply into the realm of Self-help and spirituality. I journaled, tried meditation, and practiced focusing my thoughts on gratitude, empowerment, and Self-discovery. This was all long before the current cultural glut of life coaching programs, and these small steps were revolutionary strides in my growing ability to look into my Self to find the change I needed.

Following my internal navigation system made the decision to divorce much simpler than it otherwise would have been. I was finally ready to embrace my freedom. For me, that meant changing out the scenery and the cast of characters that had surrounded me for my entire life.

When I looked around, everyone I knew seemed to be unhappy. My family seemed constantly miserable and dissatisfied. My friends spent all their time dissecting the confusion, stress, and struggle in their own lives, or else trying in vain to fix each other's problems.

It seemed so odd to me that everyone felt so challenged in their lives, no matter how successful they were, yet everything wrong in their life was someone else's fault—their spouse, their boss, their parents, their children. We were all relatively healthy and wealthy, but never once did our conversations focus on what made us happy. We were all intelligent and well-educated, but we somehow couldn't figure our way out of situations that dissatisfied us.

Of course, I understand now how normalizing this kind of conversation is. With the exception of idealistic college students or starry-eyed people who have just fallen in love, bitching and moaning is standard conversational currency in our world today. When someone comes along and proclaims how happy they are with their lives, most people will humor them to their face, then gossip about them as soon as they leave.

Essentially, we spend our social lives commiserating with each other. That's the accepted thing to do. They say misery loves company, but I think it's even more true that company loves misery. When we're disconnected from our path in life, the only thing that makes it a little more tolerable is knowing that everybody else is just as lost as we are.

THE TURNING POINT

It was starting to dawn on me with each fresh realization that my true Self was the purpose of my life, and living in integrity with my Self was the path to my happiness and fulfillment. This was very different from the societally-prescribed one I had been following. I gave up rigorous workouts and started taking hip-hop classes. Instead of kvetching with girlfriends about our terrible relationships, I spent my weekends at art museums or dancing the night away at clubs. I even gave up my food obsession and learned to obsess over something else—shopping at designer boutiques, which became my addiction of choice.

Fortunately, I had the budget to support my expensive new habit. Although I'd transitioned into a new industry, I was distinguishing myself through the same leadership qualities. Technically, I was a sales manager for a medical technology company. On a functional level, though, I was an employee development wizard. Any department I showed up in, any meeting I attended, instantly became an incubator for personal development. Somehow, I always found my way to the human heart of any obstacle and was able to help people connect the dots from their highest Self to their highest performance. When it came to sales, I could walk into a room of folded arms and leave with everyone high-fiving each other for choosing to purchase my company's product.

I was great at my job. But I was starting to wonder whether the job was great for me.

Despite my personal focus on human potential, I was still working for a medical corporation, one of the highest bullshit-per-capita industries in the game. We sold a particular product that, like any medical technology, was rapidly becoming obsolete. Each person's professional success was directly tied to pushing an agenda that was ultimately based on a lie.

I tried to tell myself that my work was valuable—after all, for patients in the hospital, I played a vital part in the healing process. I also had daily evidence that my approach to management was helping the people I worked with, enriching their lives, and helping them pursue their highest Self.

Once again, I'd gone into "fixer" mode, telling my Self that it was more important for me to be there for others than to live in integrity.

But my internal navigation system had come too far to let me stay there. Every conference call I participated in illuminated the situation for me with increasing clarity. We were all colluding in a massive lie that our work was meaningful. We said we wanted the best for the patient, but we knew that what we had to offer wasn't genuinely the best. We told doctors that we cared about people, but we knew that what we really cared about was high sales numbers. We said during meetings that we had each other's backs, but we knew that really being supportive would have meant encouraging one another to find a new job.

I guess one day my internal navigation system had had enough. I signed off yet another conference call and began to shake my head over the bullshit-fest it had been, when something inside me said, "Wake up, Tracy! You're exactly the same as them—a big freaking liar. You're lying about the product you sell, you're lying about the reason you're in this job, and you're lying about who you really are."

Then, for good measure, my internal navigation gave me one more kick in the pants: "Is it any wonder that all the men you date lie, cheat, and betray you?"

It was the first time I'd ever thought of it this way: that the world gives us back exactly what we put into it. I spent most of my life lying to others about who I was and what was important to me. If I suffered from having other people lie to me, how was that anything but fair? Call it karma, call it the law of attraction, or call it whatever you want—by presenting my Self to the world as a person who could not be trusted, I was constantly being "matched," romantically and professionally, with people whom I could not trust. If I wanted to find people worthy of being trusted, I would have to become one of those people.

This was a principle I'd already seen in play. During my years of eating disorders and twisted relationships, it seemed that most of my lifelong friends were over-focused on weight and felt dissatisfied in their romantic lives. As I grew in connection to things that mattered positively to me, I fit in less with people who were focused on the negative aspects of their lives.

When I consciously listened to myself and moved to New York, I became friends with people who, like me, were determined to make the most of their lives. The more time I spent with people who shared my love of culture, art, professional achievement, and personal improvement, the more of my Self I was able to express.

The fulfillment I felt through this evolution created a stark contrast with the areas of continued struggle in my life. But it also renewed my determination to persevere in connecting with more of my purpose and potential. As I learned new ways to work on my Self, I shared it all with my friends, who came to depend on me for advice in everything from their love lives to their careers to, yes, their ever-present thoughts.

However, even though we all enjoyed stylish, successful lives that rivaled *Sex and the City* for sheer fabulousness, our get-togethers over brunch or cocktails inevitably turned into discussions of relationship "tactics" and magic diet/exercise programs. No matter how enviable our lives looked from the outside, we still didn't feel completely happy in our own skin.

I realized that what I believed about my Self had a direct impact on the kind of people I would connect to. By living in integrity, my practical path would lead me into relationships with people who were equally connected to their own purpose and potential. I didn't need to go find new friends. By upgrading the way I approached not just my life but the way I talked about my life, then my friends would either be transformed or fall away.

Whatever level of care I gave my Self, the universe gave

more of the same. (That, I had to admit, was a pretty amazing level of support.)

That was the day I made my decision. I wasn't going to waste another minute waiting for someone or something else to make me complete. Instead, I was going to create a relationship with my Self that was so loving, so truthful, so full of care and curiosity and wonder, that it would outweigh any relationship I'd ever been in before.

I'd always known that life had to be simpler than everyone around me made it seem. I'd never been able to buy into the philosophy that suffering was the only way to grow as a person or connect to a deeper purpose. For the first time, I saw that the path to fulfilling my potential led not outward, but inward. As that inward awareness grew, it would be effortlessly expressed in action. Connecting to my true Self was the key to creating positive change in my own life and in the lives of everyone around me.

No longer would I treat my Self like a neglectful boyfriend—ignoring my needs, belittling my feelings, acting as though I didn't deserve this or that, and then splurging on a pair of designer jeans so I'd forget all the harm I'd done to my Self. Instead, I was going to prioritize my own needs and wishes, conduct my inner monologue with kindness and respect, and find out just how interesting a person that person inside me really was.

That's how 2006 became the year I truly met my Self.

MEETING MY SELF AT LAST

You know how when you first start dating someone, you notice all the little details about them? That's how my relationship with my Self began. I started paying attention to the things that made my heart thrill with joy, the things that sparked my curiosity and, above all, the things that caused me pain. If I woke up with a headache, I asked myself why. If I found myself getting cranky or weepy, I took a few minutes to check in and see what my Self was trying to communicate to me.

It didn't take long to start seeing patterns. The way I dreaded getting up early wasn't a matter of being lazy; it was something my body genuinely hated, and for which it would inevitably punish me by making me irritable or agitated throughout the day, more reactive, and more sensitive to stress. Then there was the way I felt grumpy and exhausted at the thought of going to the gym and doing the same old workout classes, making my rounds at the same old exercise machines. But I felt energized and happy after a ninety-minute dance class. And let's not forget how I was on top of the world during a meeting with doctors and hospital administrators, but felt like total crap when they signed a contract with my company when I knew there was a better medical device for better patient outcomes.

These were clear indications of what my Self was designed for—signals from my internal navigation system as it guided me on the path to a place where just being me didn't have to be a performance or cause me so much pain.

As you might expect, none of it really came as a surprise. All these realizations had been there throughout my life; I'd simply chosen to ignore them. What did surprise me, though, was how choosing to pay attention to my internal navigation made it so easy to find the good in my past experiences. I no longer felt the need to cringe over my failed marriages or hide from unflattering photos of myself. I didn't even feel inclined to gloss over the truth when people asked about my background.

Living forward in integrity with my Self was all I needed to heal from the past. It even gave me the strength and courage to return to my roots, reconnect with my family, and relaunch my life with no regrets. For the first time, there was nothing I couldn't tackle, forgive, or find compassion for. Finding my path had made me invincible.

BECOMING A HEALER

Fast forward a few years. I was back in California, not far from where I grew up. I was still working as a medical sales rep, but I was doing it to fund my doctorate in psychology. The schedule was hectic and the studies were more challenging than anything I'd ever put my mind to. But by then, my Self had adopted my high school coach's words as a mantra, "You *got* this, Thomas." I'd never felt so motivated, knowing that every day was a step toward making a profession out of my purpose—helping others heal by talking truth to them. Not only was this a seamless expression of my Self—perfectly in line with my own purpose and potential—but it also served others in getting on the path to their own purpose and potential.

The final step in my PhD program was completing my clinical internships. After applying for several different opportunities, I got matched with a county-run women's addiction clinic. The overwhelming majority of my clients there were single mothers, addicts, and/or victims of abuse. These women had all the physical and mental health symptoms that accompany that kind of stress.

These women had heard everything—tough love, spiritual empowerment, classic clinical psychology—and nothing had made a lasting difference in their lives. I'm sure my confidence looked like youthful hubris to the people supervising my first internship. I'm even more sure that if they could have overheard what I was saying to these women in our initial sessions, they might have hustled me right out of that clinic.

I wasn't coaching these women not to use crack. I wasn't scolding them for skipping work or getting back together with the partner who beat them up. Instead, I was agreeing with them. I was saying things like, "Crack makes a lot of sense when you're in so much pain," or, "It makes sense that after CPS took your kids away, you'd be depressed and want to drink even more."

But then, I'd redirect the conversation. Instead of talking all about their pain, we'd start talking about their power. For these women, this was the first time anyone had suggested they had a good, powerful, valuable Self, let alone that living in integrity with that Self could turn their lives around. They'd been told they were powerless and their salvation lay in believing in a higher power, the only thing that could deliver them from their addictions. Never before had they been empowered through connecting to themselves. I walked them through the steps I'd taken during my first year of cultivating a relationship with my Self. It was the ideal/greatest relationship of my life, the standard that I'd set for all other relationships to come. I told them about learning to hear and being guided by the internal navigation system, using positive and assertive Self-talk, finding the things they knew to be true about themselves, and focusing on honoring those things.

Over time, these women were coming to see me with growing track records of real change—they hadn't called the abusive boyfriend back, they'd taken their medications for depression and bipolar disorder, they were cutting down on smoking and getting through substance withdrawal, they were showing up for work on time, and they were making better parenting decisions. They were experiencing small-but-steady wins by following their internal navigation system and living in integrity with themselves. It was giving them the power to get through each day better than the last.

It was powerful proof that my newly-discovered Method wasn't just a luxury for those who could afford introspection. It was a real and primal connection that could empower anyone in any walk of life.

None of this went unnoticed by my mentor, the renowned energy psychologist, Dr. Adriana Popescu. Her expertise in marrying the clinical with the spiritual was a seminal part of The Method's refinement. Just as I was completing my post-doctoral internship, she approached me with a proposition. She had just taken a job as the director of

Alta Mira, a high-end rehab center in Sausalito, and she wanted me to bring my Method to the clients there.

Exhausted from my doctoral training, I wasn't sure how ready I was to acclimate to a new work environment. But Adriana urged me to stay on my path—"Don't let being tired get in the way of where you're supposed to be." The more she told me about Alta Mira, the more I saw that she was right. Alta Mira would be the perfect place to give The Method its most rigorous field test to date. Whereas, we could only go so far with the resources at the community rehab center, the patients at Alta Mira could afford any kind of treatment they needed, from an array of recommended lab tests and other clinical evaluations to hormone replacement therapy to elite nutrition, from major career shifts to lengthy sabbaticals. There would be no limits placed on our ability to fine-tune our patients' treatment at every level.

It was time to see how far The Method could really go.

HEALING AT THE DEEPEST LEVEL

Let me tell you, being rich and powerful is no walk in the park. I was sitting in clinical sessions with business moguls, fashion models, politicians, film actors, people who flew to their sessions on private planes, people who never had to work another day in their lives, and I was hearing stories that would make your hair curl. The vast resources our patients possessed only made it easier for them to remain in denial and hurt themselves at a faster rate and a deeper level than the average person can afford.

And just like in the community rehab clinic, most of them shared a belief that things could not get better for them. They would keep spending the money on therapy because they had it, but they didn't see themselves ever losing their anger, their anxiety, or their craving for high-priced vices. The only Self they knew was a Self for whom being abstinent meant living in pain.

In a lot of ways, these patients were prisoners of their own success. They had families, companies, entourages, all hovering over them with a network of expectations. I saw that underneath each client's glamor, wealth, and power was a person completely out of touch with their true Self—or, worse, someone who knew their true Self was in there but too frightened to let that Self show. In other words, they were just like the person I used to be.

In many cases, my patients were actually the child of wealthy and powerful parents. These people would gladly have spent every penny they had if it meant seeing their son or daughter well and happy. In those situations, after just a session or two, I had to level with the parents by saying, "I can help your son or daughter heal, and they'll never shoot heroin/have a seizure/cut themselves again. But you have to be ready to let them be someone different from the person you've always expected them to be."

In the long run, every client needed the same thing from me: permission and guidance in breaking down the barriers that stood between them and the path to their purpose and full potential. Many times, it simply came down to a matter of, "I don't want to do this anymore," whether *this* meant taking a role in a movie, buying yet another palatial home, having to answer a call from or playing shrink to their mother every day, or running the company their family had built over the past ten generations. There were a lot of pissed-off producers, partners, and parents in the background, and part of my job also consisted of helping the client learn to get their loved ones on board with their choice to meet their true needs and to live their unique path.

You wouldn't believe the changes I saw take place. People who suffered from schizophrenia got off their medication. Married couples split apart by infidelity, alcoholism, and sex addiction came back together and renewed their love. People with bodies and brains ravaged by eating disorders bloomed into healthy, happy, confident humans. Best of all, these patients were able to adopt the healing technique of connecting with their internal navigation system in a way that would lead them forward on the path to fulfilling their purpose and potential.

And the craziest part was how quickly it all happened. Because these people could afford every kind of therapy imaginable, we were able to apply The Method at every level of their physical, mental, and spiritual being. Their unlimited resources meant they could instantly respond to any kind of guidance from their internal navigation system—they could instantly quit a job they hated, purchase an arsenal of elite nutritional supplements, or access every kind of evaluation that I deemed essential to getting to the root of their hidden addiction-causing factors.

As a result, I got to see in real time what happens when the internal navigation system is allowed free reign over a person's life. What happens is nothing short of miraculous. I saw The Method bring people off suicide watch. Lonely people found love. People paralyzed by bitterness, pain, codependence, and fear got out there and made productive choices in their lives. And there were virtually no relapses.

THE METHOD COMES BACK TO ME

There's no doubt that watching The Method prove itself

at Alta Mira was tremendously satisfying to me. But it was also an occasion for me to reflect on my own internal navigation once again. I knew that the path to my purpose and potential ultimately lay with having my own clinical practice where I could teach The Method on my own terms.

In the end, what made me effective was my ability to exemplify The Method for others. They trusted me because they could see how much I trusted my Self. If I was to ignore my own internal navigation, even if it was in the service of helping others, my power would be gone. How could my patients learn to trust their internal navigation if I was ignoring my own?

Once I started my private therapeutic coaching practice, word spread even more quickly than it had at Alta Mira. Eventually, I brought together a team of therapists and trained them to support my rapidly growing practice.

Following The Method has led me into an amazing professional life. I've built a successful company on the basis of being my Self—using my most intuitive skills to treat people all over the world through my virtual coaching company. I've traveled all over the world, both for pleasure and going to conferences and workshops. I've collaborated with people of incredible resources in the service of helping others find the path to living their purpose and potential.

But that's just the beginning. The Method has also continued to transform my personal life. My physical health has bloomed thanks to a passion for yoga and ballroom dancing. I've led my family in redesigning our relationships in a way that lets us enjoy each other while respecting our differences. I'm now married to a man who couldn't be more perfect for me if I'd designed him myself.

Finally, The Method has also allowed me to see my own story in a new way. I look back on everything I've described in this chapter with feelings of empathy and even gratitude. I see with absolute clarity that nobody in my life was ever trying to hurt me. In fact, they were usually trying to love me in the best way they knew how, while dealing with their own disconnection from Self. Ultimately, the pain that we endured was instrumental in leading me to create The Method. In turn, The Method has allowed me to help my own family, along with countless others, overcome pain by finding the path to their purpose and potential. What could have ended as trauma and brokenness has now become the opportunity to be a force of good in the world—how can I be anything but grateful for that?

Following The Method held me to a high standard of accountability, especially where my "healer" tendency is concerned. It's kind of a catch-22—I believe The Method can help everybody, but the only way I can faithfully convey it to others is by following The Method myself. My ability to offer healing to anyone starts with recognizing that I can't personally heal everyone. Helping others to heal themselves comes from using myself as The Method that they absorb as the antithesis of the negative aspects/dysfunctional aspects of what they absorbed from their parents' relationship with themselves.

However, my internal navigation system has brought me too far for me to stop trusting it now. I've learned that every time life brings me up against a limitation, by leaning even more into The Method of the relationship with my Self, I create a new opportunity for living my purpose and experiencing potential every day. The book you're reading right now would never have come about if my internal navigation hadn't made me recognize my own limitations as a one-on-one healer.

No matter what made you pick up this book—a desire to heal from pain, a last-ditch effort to overcome lifelong challenges, a suspicion that you have yet to reach your full potential—I am delighted for you to discover The Method for your Self. Following your internal navigation system is a lifelong adventure. Even if you and I never get to meet, from now on we'll be on this adventure side by side, discovering the practical path to living our purpose and potential, one day and one moment at a time.

Chapter Four

REFINING AND SIMPLIFYING THE METHOD

There are teachers and then there are guides. For every ten people who offer you perfectly valid insight, there might be only one whose words truly resonate with you on a profound level. While insight is great, it cannot do the work for you. Creating a great relationship with your Self *is* what makes living your purpose and potential a very practical process. The practical process of living in integrity with yourself creates the clarity of your purpose that allows you to experience the fulfillment of all your potential.

One of the first things your internal navigation does for

you is attract you toward the teachings that can get you started on the path to knowing your purpose and experiencing your potential in each moment of your life. Your navigation is no elitist—it doesn't care what the teacher's credentials are, whether they are perched on an academic pedestal or live in the same house as you, whether other people respect them or make fun of them. Your internal navigation system knows what it needs and, when you tune into that, it leads you down a path that feels right for you. Once it finds a person or an ideology that can put those needs into words, your navigation will take every useful thing those teachers can offer you.

In the previous chapter, I shared the story of how The Method played out in my life. But I don't want you to think any of it happened in a vacuum. I created my path by building off the teachings of a number of wise people. Their insights were instrumental in helping me build the practical framework that I'm sharing with you in this book.

In this chapter, I'm going to show you how my internal navigation not only drew me toward these teachings, but also how it helped me interpret and apply these teachings as I connected with my Self at the deepest levels, discovered my purpose, and began living at more of my potential. In sharing these stories, my hope is twofold: First, that you'll have an added wealth of resources that can help you on your quest toward healing. But also, that you'll have an example of how to be a student while still being in integrity with your Self.

When you're suffering deeply, it is very easy to become a devoted disciple of one specific teacher, practice, or ideology. It may be an outflow of a tendency to addiction, or it may simply be that you've finally found something that relieves your pain, and you're clinging to it like a drowning person to a life raft.

But you'll find as you grow that your internal navigation system wants its freedom even while being taught. Giving your Self this freedom is essential to assimilating a teaching in a way that yields the most benefit. Your internal navigation system needs you to trust your Self first and foremost. This foundational trust of your Self is the only way you can safely trust anyone or anything else.

Without allowing your internal navigation system to reveal to you what you're drawn to, any teaching, no matter how effective, will create a "drag" effect on your personal growth. Worst case scenario, you'll be more vulnerable to abuse from teachers who care more about building a following than helping their followers. It is important to distinguish your relationship to those teachings from the relationship you have with the teachers.

It's equally important to remember that our teachers are seldom our gurus for life. The last thing I ever want for my clients is to depend on me indefinitely. My job as a psychologist is to give you a complete set of tools to connect to your purpose and experience the fulfillment of your potential that most people are craving. I expect my office, virtual or otherwise, to be a revolving door, because patients are quickly and effectively empowered to lead themselves and be their own healer. That's what The Method is all about.

I've had the good fortune to personally meet and interact with some of the most advanced spiritual advisors, therapists, and leaders. (One of them even gave me her shoes...but more about that later.) My connection to those people runs deep, because I will be forever grateful for their help in finding my path. But that connection was able to remain strong precisely because my internal navigation was always in charge of how I applied their teachings. When my navigation guided me to move beyond a specific teaching or practice and on to the next one that could serve me, I followed its guidance without hesitation. When it told me to improvise and make what they recommend into my very own version of their instruction, I listened and lived the collaboration of their Self and my Self as cocreators of something with even greater potential than either of us might've managed on our own.

It goes without saying that that's what I want for you as you read this book.

Ultimately, no teacher can convey anything to you that your internal navigation system doesn't already know. The essential good of a teacher is to offer modes of articulation and practice that serve as signposts on your unique path through life. The heart of the process is through a resonance that something we say connects you and awakens you to even more of your Self that wants to be alive.

THE LAUNCHING POINT—OPRAH

As it was for so many people in the 1980s, Oprah Winfrey was my introduction to Self-help. What set her program apart from other talk shows of that time was her willingness to be vulnerable about her own issues—from struggling with weight to surviving sexual assault. She's really the original when it comes to authentic, unscripted vulnerability on TV, and that allowed her to get real with her guests and her audience in a way that nobody else had done. I don't know that Oprah gets enough credit for the bravery that led her to do this. It says a lot about her own internal navigation system; I think that's why my own internal navigation responded to her teaching and modeling of authentic humanity so eagerly.

I started watching *The Oprah Winfrey Show* with my

grandmother when I was fifteen. By my twenties, I was religiously taping the show on my VCR. Her show might as well have been my church. At Oprah's suggestion, I began journaling about my experiences, thoughts, and feelings. This gave me my very first opportunity to experience the "observer" in action, though I didn't know that's what it was at the time. This experience became fascinating to me—who was that person looking back at me from the pages of my notebook? Some people struggle with Self-consciousness when they journal; not me. I think my internal navigation was so glad to have this outlet that it never occurred to me to hold back or cover up potentially embarrassing revelations. I experienced the benefit of journaling in its purest form, and I continued the practice well into my thirties and all the way through to today. I start the day with journaling gratitude, what I'm accomplishing, and what my vision is for my life...and I see what comes up.

The second gift Oprah gave me was the intentional practice of gratitude. For me, this became so much more than simply focusing on positives over negatives. It was a portal to becoming intensely, intimately conscious of my Self. Whenever I think of New York City's Central Park, I'm taken back to the mornings I spent running on the various trails, timing each footfall to a new source of gratitude, from the sunlight on my hair, to the strength in my feet, to the endorphins that rushed through my blood, to the skyline that loomed over the trees, reminding me of what a glorious city I lived in.

The more my gratitude increased, so did my awareness of what I was feeling and where it found expression in my body, my brain, and my emotions. This was the launching point for me to continue to seek opportunities to learn from as many teachers as possible. Most of those I connected to in my early years were through the Oprah show, as she showcased a continuous and multifaceted crop of inspirational people.

THE ULTIMATE PAIN RELIEF—WILLIAMSON, TOLLE, AND DR. PHIL

Like so many people, I encountered the new wave of spirituality writing with some skepticism. When my mother sent me the book, *Return to Love* by Marianne Williamson, with its claim to offer a "course in miracles," my first thought was, "Are you kidding me?"

Although I wasn't sure about this course in miracles concept, my internal navigation system guided me to crack open the book, just to see what it had to offer. Within those pages, I immediately fastened on the cue for what would become the first tenet of The Method.

Marianne taught that the only thing that's missing from

any situation is what you're not bringing to it. Her premise was that anything that frustrates you about someone else is symptomatic, not of something lacking in them, but of something lacking in your Self that you're not bringing forward. This teaching was my first clue that a relationship with my Self was foundational for any other relationship I would have.

Eckhart Tolle's *The Power of Now* built upon this principle. His concept of the "observer" allowed me to get outside my own head and address the frustrations borne of personal weakness and insufficiency in a nonjudgmental way. Once I mastered it, observance became my ultimate form of pain relief.

Tolle also instilled the understanding of Selfhood as a practice. It was revolutionary to me to consider that the Self is the product of intention, commitment, and habituation. The only difference between the unhappy, pain-filled Self and the happy, potential-filled Self is that the first one is learned before we know that we're learning it. Unless our parents and authority figures are exceptionally evolved people, connection with our true Self is a gift we must give ourselves.

If Marianne gave me the first principle, and Tolle gave me the means to administer it, the final leg of the table was modality, and that came from Dr. Phil. I immediately liked him when he began showing up on Oprah's show as a featured guest—his avuncular persona, his folksy southern accent, but, above all, his compassion paired with uncompromising candor. Some of the teachers I'd been studying up to that point delivered their teaching from an intellectual or spiritual distance. But Dr. Phil reminded me of my high school coach—he came off like a friend who loved you too much to let you get away with being anything less than your best. Calling myself out became comical and amusing, which allowed me to make consciousness as fun as it needed to be for it to be practical for me. Fun is a huge requirement for me to feel the fulfillment my Self longs for.

The combined effect of these three teachers has really made me the transformational strategist I am today. My grasp of pain as being predicated on what people perceive within allows me to intuit a lot about patients beyond the experiences they share with me. My personal practice of observance helps me ground each patient in nonjudgmental reality. Finally, I'm known for never letting diplomacy get the better of my desire to see people connect to their truth, which will be the only productive path they can walk down. I will always "go there" with my clients.

Geneen Roth's books were all pivotal in my gradual recovery from my obsession with food, dieting, losing weight and my body. *Women, Food and God* was seminal to the last stage of complete and total freedom from this dysfunctional relationship with food and my Self-image. I know I'm not alone in that experience; her book helped thousands of women see the deeper roots of their issues around food. But her last book also gave me an entry point to start doing "check-ins" with my internal navigation system.

Geneen's genius lies in reintroducing intuitive eating. For generations of women, the primal practice of eating had been warped and twisted within a cultural power play designed to keep them docile. Her books have offered detailed, step-by-step guidance in how to reconnect with the many different appetites germane to being human, and how to distinguish physical hunger from other kinds of hunger.

I adopted and practiced her eating protocol religiously and immediately expanded it to literally every aspect of my life as I began to check in and connect to my Self more than ever before. She helped me reengage with my body's natural rhythms and release the fear that I could not be trusted when it comes to food or living even more of my truth. I learned for myself which foods my body responds well to, which foods didn't have much to offer me in terms of pleasure or fuel, and what kind of intervals my body needed to process the food I ate. I became acquainted for the first time with what it feels like to be both present and nourished, and I began to see them as the same thing. I also began to experience the amazing joy of being the person who offers my Self the nourishment it needs.

One of Geneen's most famous concepts from her books, says, "Our relationship to food is our relationship to Self." For me, that concept resonated deeply. I was in my twenties and had finally conquered the behavioral aspect of my eating disorder, and was at a healthy weight that nobody could find fault with either way. Still, I wasn't completely free. I could feel the constant presence of that pattern. I was simply managing the eating disorder, along with the pain that the disorder attempted to manage. I remember looking at Geneen, a glorious and wise woman at age fifty, and thinking, "I will never get that far if I don't get the freedom part." Even though I was loving my Self, I still wasn't fully tuned into my navigation. I still didn't trust my Self to make the decisions that were best for me.

The longer I practiced Geneen's food protocol, the less it became about food and the more it became about checking in with my Self. I didn't know it then, but I was beginning to experience the joy of relationship to Self. Food used to be the bone I threw to my Self in lieu of nourishing it with attention. But the more I checked in with my Self about why it wanted food, the less food became the focus and the more I was able to identify stress and release it from my system.

Geneen describes in the book how she finally realized that much of her thoughts, her energies, and her skills were going into weight management. She said, "I realized one day that my life was not meant to be on the fucking scale losing the same pounds over and over and over." You can imagine how much this resonated with me. It was like she'd held a mirror up to me. At the same time, my whole reason for focusing on food the way I did was to manage the pain I felt. It was, after all, the legacy of women in my family.

If my internal navigation was directing me toward focusing on food and eating as a way to manage my pain, I had to lean into that. It was, as Geneen taught, important to check in about physical versus psychological hunger. But I believed it was just as important to check in about where the discomfort was coming from. So, when I would eat according to Geneen's protocol, I would carefully observe the feelings that rose up—the impulse to refill my plate before I'd finished the first helping, the urge to get up and turn on the TV rather than focusing on the tastes in my mouth. I saw how my Self never wanted to stay in a moment of pleasure, relaxation, or gratification for very long. It wanted to either rush to overindulgence or else move on to other activities it could abuse. In other words, it was looking for opportunities to be in a familiar form of pain. It was looking for ways to avoid being with the perceived empty Self. Eating seemed to temporarily fill up the false nothingness that in my disconnection to Self, seemed very real.

Noticing that tendency allowed me to make the choice to sit still, to stay in the tension until it passed. Pressing through those moments of internal discomfort forced me to see that food was nothing more than the metaphor for giving the Self what it wants, what it needs, and trusting it to know what is best. The longer I practiced this, the more I saw that I could trust my Self to tell me when to stop eating, and it would be easy. I could actually see the difference between what I really needed and what I perceived I needed. That was a critical nuance that changed everything. The more I practiced this with food, the more I saw it play out in every other aspect of my life. My Self just needed to taste freedom in this one area in order to give it a hunger for full, holistic freedom.

THE IMPORTANCE OF LANGUAGE—BYRON KATIE

I remember actually telling Geneen at one of her workshops that if she didn't hurry up and parlay her intuitive eating principles into a book about intuitive living, I was going to write that book myself. But, of course, that book already existed—it was *Loving What Is: Four Questions That Can Change Your Life,* and Geneen's own books make frequent reference to the author, Byron Katie.

Even though Geneen credits Byron in her books, for me, Byron picked up where Geneen left off. While working at a halfway house for women with severe eating disorders, Byron developed a therapy known as The Work. The Work's central tenet can be expressed in a quotation, which has become a mantra among Byron's followers: "I love my thoughts. I'm just not tempted to believe them."

The theme of her work and writing is that whatever story you're telling yourself, you have to be wary of putting 100 percent faith in its accuracy. A lot of our pain comes from telling ourselves stories about what happened to us, what people feel about us, and what it all means. Byron's work with clients involves asking them to consider how they know any given thought or story is true, examining their response to the thought, and imagining how their lives would be different if the thought or story were not a part of it.

For me, taking these ideas to heart meant taking every thought captive as it showed up. Not just the ones about the story of my past, or my identity in the present, but even things as small as the inbox on my desk or my plans for the weekend. And thanks to Byron's emphasis on the power of words, I became rigorously accurate in the language I used about my thoughts, especially in the moments of checking in with my internal navigation system.

If I was feeling stressed at work, for example, I would check in and ask my Self what I was feeling. The observer would answer with something like this: "I'm feeling stressed because I have to get all this paperwork filed right now." But then, Byron's accuracy principle would show up: "Do you really *have* to get it *all* done right *now?*" When you come right down to it, that thought was entirely inaccurate. Of course, I didn't have to get it done right then. It was on my task list, and I wanted to get it done quickly, but if I was being strictly honest, that wasn't the answer to the original check-in question anyway. The true answer was more like this: "I'm feeling anxious that this job is going to take too long for me to leave work when I was planning to."

The benefit of this rigorously accurate language started with how I was able to handle stress. It has an amazing way of stopping small issues from escalating into the pain that blocks us from our potential. But it also had an amazing effect on the people around me. When I started to speak more accurately to others, they started to speak more accurately to me.

This gave me an idea. What if, instead of only being strictly accurate in things related to me alone, I was also strictly accurate in the way I talked about things that related to others? When I was asked to put in extra hours at work to complete a task, instead of giving a long-winded explanation about why I couldn't (or shouldn't have to), I'd simply say, "I'll be available to do that on Monday." And guess what? Speaking this way totally changed the dynamic of the conversation.

Byron Katie showed me that when you limit your talk to what you actually have evidence for, you spare yourself and others an enormous amount of pain. So many of the things we say have stress layered into them, from, "I need to empty the dishwasher," to "I should have listened to my mother." Whether we speak these thoughts aloud or simply act on them, their presence only serves to multiply the stress in the world. The body hears words like "need to" or "should have" as danger signals. They induce what I call "everyday PTSD," a type of terrorizing of ourselves that is so common, few people even notice it. But as we've talked about already, those danger signals simply were not accurate. As such, they were impractical. All they did was take me out of the potential of each moment I was living in.

I saw that by speaking kindly and truthfully to my Self, I could not only sidestep all the pain and stress, but I could bring myself right back to making those moments full of potential. The more I did it, the more my path opened up to not only change my own life, but to change the world around me.

EMBRACING THE SELF—ADYASHANTI

I first met the Zen teacher Adyashanti as my neighbor in the Bay Area, speaking a block away from my office in Marin. He was (and still is) famous for the *satsangs* he would hold at his home—spiritual gatherings where people could discuss, teach, and be taught, or simply enjoy the company of fellow seekers. I was instantly drawn to him, because unlike so many spiritual teachers, he was hilariously funny. So often at these *satsangs*, he would sit among his admirers in silence, only to open his mouth with an off-the-wall observation that broke the otherworldly reverence and made everyone instant friends.

Being able to interact directly with Adyashanti as well as read his books had a similar effect on me as an individual. Many of the things he said were distillations of what I'd learned from previous writers and teachers, but knowing the person behind them as my neighbor and friend allowed me to internalize those teachings in a new way. His writing stemmed from his own experience of realizing, after fourteen years of studying Zen, that he was the Buddha he had been looking for. This experience was what allowed him to stop being Steven Gray and to embrace a new identity—because it was, in truth, not a new identity, but one that he'd been all along.

Adyashanti asserts that it's okay to leave behind the stories that we carry around—a task that even those who have suffered the most sometimes loath to do. It's understandable that when you've worked so hard to overcome the pain, trauma, and stress in your life, you'd kind of want to keep that work as part of your story, like a medal you've won in a war. Maybe you even need to keep picking at those scars, reopening those wounds, insisting on more pain in your story. If so, it's probably for one simple reason: it makes you feel alive, because to not identify with painful stories can feel like a literal physical death...the kind of psychological death that can feel like insanity. You don't know how to be okay with just being okay—checking in and feeling your organs working, your breath sustaining you, your pulse keeping pace.

Adyashanti points out that most of us learn our Self-concept through stress. This is given to us by our parents as we grow up. You have to share with your sister; you have to eat your vegetables; you have to go to college; you have to put yourself out there. Layered on top of that is the world's response to you, which you naturally assume is based off your performance of those fundamental duties. By the time you reach adulthood, you know who you are based off what you've done, how well you've done it, and how it affected other people.

It's incredibly rare that anyone lives their full life without some negative feedback, even when they were doing what they were taught to do. Say you heeded your parents' admonition to work hard at school, so you could get a good job and be able to support a family someday. You wanted that, so you threw yourself into studying. You had friends, but you were known as a nerd. You internalized that identity along with its classic corollary: girls don't like you because you're a nerd. Now, it's twenty years later. You have the family you always wanted, but you still have that story of "girls don't like me" paired with the story that your parents gave you about how important it is to work hard. Those two stories have helped you build a new story with a terrible conflict: you have to work hard at your job to take care of your wife who doesn't like you because you're a nerd who works hard at your job.

At this point, it doesn't even matter whether it's true or not that your wife doesn't like you, or whether your job is nerdy, or whether you have to work hard at it. You're operating according to those stories because that's all you know about who you are. You could go to marriage counseling or get a different job, but the story would still be hovering over you because without it...there's no *you*.

When you realize how stories can compound on each other, it's easy to see how people can end up resorting to extreme behaviors like abandoning their families, living a double life, or even committing suicide. They don't realize they are literally trapped in a false "reality," and they believe the only escape is to throw everything away. The only thing more frightening than the horrible reality they live in is the emptiness they feel without it.

Learning this through Adyashanti's teaching and his book, *Falling into Grace*, I realized that if I was going to let go of my pain story and the Self-harmful behaviors that accompanied it, I had to be comfortable in a state of not yet knowing what the real story was. I had to let life happen to me without supplying the context, and just let it be. I had to stop fearing the emptiness that wasn't there. If I felt my actual Self, there was substance...the furthest thing from emptiness. I was solid as a physical being and there was so much fullness that emptiness now seemed laughable.

I confess that I felt a little trepidation when I set out to practice this "emptiness." But what truly shocked me was how *good* it felt. When I allowed myself to be a vessel just for experience, I felt my Self awakening inside me (just like Adyashanti said it would). In the absence of a pain story, I felt the actual physical sensation of my body recalibrating. It was like my Self was standing up tall for the first time, flexing its muscles, stretching its wings. By emptying myself of stressful narratives, I felt for the first time in my life that I was full. By discovering how interesting it was to check in with my Self, I proved that the emptiness I feared was false.

I remember thinking, "My god, what a revelation." I didn't need pain to feel like my Self. Pain had been taking up so much space inside me, but now since it's gone, I am filled with the fullness of my true Self.

COMING FULL CIRCLE

As The Method began to take shape in my life, it continually brought me back to Oprah's guidance. While I was learning, growing, and embodying The Method, she was shifting away from the celebrity gossip model and leaning into her own quest for spiritual, intellectual, and physical health. She was differentiating herself as the leader and curator of thought leaders, and I was eating it up—journaling, practicing gratitude, and recording her shows on the DVR, so I could binge-watch them on the weekends.

The importance Oprah played in my life is wonderfully illustrated by this story. It's one of my favorite stories to share, both for what it says about Oprah and what it taught me about my Self.

Fast forward to Harpo Studios. Melissa was seated in the front row, alongside a slew of other guests who were going to talk about the whole working vs. stay-at-home mother topic.

I was seated a few rows back, mostly in the company of the husbands of the women who were guests. As usual, I was chatting with everyone around me, making friends. But we all burst into cheers as Oprah entered the studio. As the crew got set up for the first segment, she chatted with the audience, asked us how we were doing, and then she confessed she wasn't doing so hot at that moment—her shoes were killing her.

"My assistant is going to be the death of me," she grumbled good-naturedly. "She knows I wear a size up in Jimmy Choos—these are a nine but I need a ten." We all commiserated with her until the crew signaled that they were ready. Oprah took the stage, and the first segment went live on the air.

After a few commercial breaks where Oprah kept making fun of her feet-hurting shoes, it was time for the taping of "Oprah After the Show." But in between the last segment and the next round of segments for the aftershow, Oprah kicked the shoes off and said, "That's it, I can't take these damned Jimmy Choos anymore." I leaned over to the people sitting next to me and said, "You know, the funny thing is that those shoes are worth about $3,000, and after today, they're going to get tossed in a closet or donated to Goodwill."

The taping was about to start up again, but I couldn't focus, because now the gears in my mind were spinning. *Those Jimmy Choos will never see the light of day again...I've always wanted some Jimmy Choos...it just happens that I'm also a size 9.* When the next commercial break came and Oprah started to grumble again about the shoes, my hand spontaneously flew up in the air and I piped up, loud and clear, "I'll take them!"

Melissa told me later that she didn't even need to turn around—she knew there was only one person in the whole room who would have said something like that. But everybody else wheeled around in their seats, shocked by the audacity of somebody volunteering to adopt Oprah's $3,000 high heels.

Oprah scanned the audience until she locked eyes with

me. Shoes in hand, she started up the aisle to where I was sitting. She was saying, "No way these will fit you—you're petite, your feet will be too small." I insisted, "No, no—I'm a size nine, just like you," and I kicked my foot right up into the air, as if I were Cinderella.

And Oprah, without batting an eye, held the shoe up to my foot like Prince Charming. Sure enough, it was a match. Placing the Jimmy Choos into my eager arms, she said, "They're all yours." Over her shoulder, she told the audience, "You've got to ask for what you want in life."

Of course, everyone started laughing and clapping, loving the spontaneous display of the outrageous generosity that Oprah is known for. But for me, it went a lot deeper than that.

I hadn't come to the show looking for a way to interact with Oprah. Even when I started thinking about what would happen to the shoes, I hadn't planned out what to say or when to say it—the words just leapt out of my mouth. After years of connecting with Oprah and her teachings, my internal navigation simply knew that she would appreciate my audacity, that she would respond well to someone asking for what they wanted, that our shared energy for life would cause us to connect.

There are a lot of times where I've loved my navigation

and the way it directs me through life, but that episode was truly a high point. That brief interaction with Oprah made me fall so deeply in love with my internal navigation, not only for the way it scored me a fabulous pair of shoes, but for how my navigation had created this practical path to meeting the teacher who had helped me discover it.

Asking for what you want in life...what could be more practical than that?

YOU ARE THE PRACTICAL PATH

Ultimately, each of us is our own teacher. We won't connect to any idea, concept, or practice unless our internal navigation calls us to it. In creating an incredible relationship with your Self, you create your unique practical path through life. The role of any teacher is to affirm those discoveries and help you articulate, clarify, and simplify the path to your purpose so you can live your potential.

Never forget that you will and should have your own version of every useful tool you learn. This is what is meant by saying, "You *are* the practical path." Making every lesson your own will serve your teachers by mirroring the principles they have taught back to them. Through you, they will see the true effect of what they are offering the world, and if they are wise, they will use what you teach them to refine it.

Remembering this will help you maintain a healthy balance in your relationship to teachers. When it comes to connecting with your Self, your purpose, and living your full potential, you are as important to your teachers as they are to you.

Chapter Five

MAKING THE COMMITMENT TO YOUR SELF

———

I still remember the first time I saw her.

Let's call her Jane.

She was the poster child for Self-abuse. Years of alcoholism had left her face haggard beyond her age. Ongoing anorexia caused her joints to creak audibly, yet, she still exercised compulsively for fear of excess calories sticking to her skeletal frame. She was on multiple medications for a host of mysterious allergies; she constantly fell into relationships with manipulative, emotionally distant men; and credit card debt from compulsive shopping had put her into a financial chokehold. But the most chilling thing about her was the way her eyes stared vacantly out of her emaciated face. It was like looking into the window of a dilapidated house—there appeared to be nobody inside. But, because I knew my true Self intimately, it allowed me to become even more able to connect to the healthy Self living inside all my clients. I could see the core being I knew I was to create a relationship with...from my true Self to hers; that was where my focus would lie.

Looking at her, I thought, "This is where The Method is going to prove itself at the most epic level."

I'd seen The Method break the power of narcotic and opioid addiction, depolarize personalities, fuse shattered marriages back together, and rekindle creative inspiration that was D.O.A. But something about Jane's case struck me as being altogether one of a kind.

This woman's Self wasn't just fractured—it had been ground into powder. She'd given up on her Self to such an extent that even her internal organs were taking the signal and beginning to shut down.

Flash forward a month later; Jane looks like a different person. Her skin is positively glowing. Her body looks healthy. Her demeanor is alert and energetic. But the most amazing thing isn't her appearance. It's the way she looks *at* people. When you meet her eyes, you see a person looking back at you—someone with emotions, opinions, and a vibrant will to live. At last, there is a Self that is emerging to the forefront.

COMMITMENT IS CENTRAL

Why did The Method work for Jane in a way that no other therapy had?

The first reason was that she'd been pushed to the breaking point. She'd been taking on more and more stress throughout her life, until her body had no choice but to shut down. Despite the emotional and mental disorders that plagued her, her inner will to live was finally calling for a change.

Still, plenty of people in pain reach this point and choose not to turn around, but instead, they forge ahead into darkness. In a lot of ways, Jane fit the profile of someone whose despair would prevent her from trusting me—just another health professional whom her family had brought in to save her.

This is where the second and more powerful reason comes in. The Method worked for Jane because it was *hers*. I put the tools in her hands and encouraged her to listen and commit to her Self. This was the one thing she had never tried. The idea that she was enough, that she had everything she needed to recover her Self, created just enough curiosity to get her on the path to connecting with her purpose and potential.

At times, clients would want to make their successful treatment about me—what I said, how I listened, how different my approach was from other therapists they'd seen. Don't get me wrong, I love hearing people say that I was the only one to make a radical difference in their lives. Nothing fulfills me like seeing somebody acknowledge my help in their healing process. However, as I always remind them, giving me credit for their healing is deflecting from the power of their own internal navigation system. My job is simply to show them that their internal navigation system exists and encourage them to listen to it.

The whole point of The Method is that you are a Self-healing entity. You become your own physician and you heal thy Self. You are the one to lead yourself down the path to living your purpose and experiencing your full potential.

All I do for my clients—and for you as the reader of this book—is what we talked about in the previous chapter:

articulate the truths that your internal navigation system already knows. In all honesty, though, this articulation piece is just icing on the cake. Your internal navigation system has everything it needs to transform your life today.

Everything, that is, except commitment from you.

GET READY TO GET WEIRD

Why do you think people find it so hard to commit, in general? It's because we're so used to taking external cues from the world. Our conditioning makes us respond to whatever triggers or cues hit us in the right nature-and-nurture spot.

Most therapy follows that same pattern. Just like Jane, people go to providers expecting to trade one set of expectations for another and end up projecting all of their relationship patterns onto the provider who, if they aren't conscious, will also do the same back to the client and become another obstacle in the client's attempts to feel whole. Along with sifting through the minutiae of your past for reasons why you are the way you are, one of the most tired tropes of therapy is the "homework" concept. Odds are good that you've had a therapist give you assignments to better yourself in various ways—meditation exercises, food diaries, having conversations with various people in your life, journaling about it all—then quizzing you about how you fulfilled all these expectations.

None of these activities are inherently unhelpful. In fact, we utilize action-based assignments outside of our sessions to facilitate consistent evolutionary progress that isn't going at a snail's pace for ten years. The problem is that if the relationship with the Self isn't the foundation of the process, the homework or recovery steps people are expected to do can be just another external mandate that unfortunately can reinforce the very problem it's seeking to solve.

You start with a person whose core issue is that she has years of expectations built up around a false, inauthentic Self. Then you complicate that person's core issue with a multitude of stresses brought on by other relationships and the expectations they place on this person. Finally, you offer that person a doctor/patient relationship that introduces a whole new set of expectations to fulfill. And that's somehow supposed to fix the issues that were caused by undue expectations in the first place?

I don't think so. Not without a solid foundation of the relationship with the Self.

Is it any wonder that the vast majority of patients drift

from one doctor to the next with no real progress? Is it any wonder that no matter what new protocol, ideology, or approach they try, their initial enthusiasm yields no practical results? I don't care if it's the best protocol in the world—if there's no buy-in from the true Self inside the patient, it won't work. And the fact is that a patient simply cannot buy into any protocol unless it translates into a practical path that stems from within their internal navigation system.

That's why I tell every patient, as soon as our session gets underway, that I am not there to dictate to them. I'm not going to reward them for following my advice or shame them for neglecting it. I tell them that their internal navigation system already knows what they need, and I'm just there to offer a safe space—a "container," I like to call it— as they learn to listen and follow their navigation. (We'll talk more about that "container" concept in Chapter 8.)

Some patients are weirded out by this at first. But at the same time, they're ready for something a little weird. They've tried every way they can think of to alleviate their suffering—medication, rehab, good old-fashioned denial, and, of course, years of traditional talk therapy. They might even be coping and gritting their teeth, one-day-at-a-time throughout their life, but they can feel themselves drowning in their own pain.

Some of these patients are in what I call their "wisdom phase" of life and are willing to give it one last try before they succumb to living out the rest of their lives in pain. Others are in a full-throttle midlife crisis, one that goes way past the panacea of a facelift or a fancy new car. But a surprising number of my patients are quite young, in their twenties or even late teens. They usually come to my office under the watchful eye of concerned parents, who take me aside before the session to share their grief and requirements of me. Not only has their beloved child broken their hearts repeatedly, but now, instead of fulfilling their potential, they'll be spending the best years of their life in therapy while their parents clean up after them.

I couldn't disagree more with this assessment. When a young person walks into my office, I am thoroughly delighted. Not for the pain they are suffering, obviously, but for the deeper reason that caused their pain to manifest. What a wonderful opportunity for them; they're going to tune in to their internal navigation system a good ten to twenty years ahead of the curve. The heartache they've been through already is nothing compared to the heartache they're going to avoid by learning to live in integrity with themselves now.

No matter what stage of life you're in, The Method works because you're ready to commit to getting out of your pain, whatever it takes.

That's good, because The Method is going to ask you to do things you never thought possible.

...But in a way, you're going to love.

PAIN = MISSED POTENTIAL

The whole reason The Method works is because it is *your* Method. It's about you cultivating a relationship with your Self where you intimately learn all the individual parts of your mind-body-spirit complex and how those parts work together.

Let me explain.

Pain is the natural result of a misalignment between what you want and what you're doing. It's the feeling that occurs whenever you miss out on living in your purpose and potential in a given moment.

It doesn't matter if you're a single working mom on welfare, or the daughter of international royalty—I've worked with patients at both ends of that spectrum as well as everyone in between. No matter what you're doing or who you're trying to be, if it's not being done in obedience to your internal navigation system, the result is pain. Pure and simple.

It doesn't even matter whether what you're doing is "good," "right" or simply "useful." If you've ever tried to reason your pain away by saying something like, "I'm just trying to be a good father," or "This happens to everyone in my position," you know from experience that your internal navigation system does not work like a Hollywood agent. It isn't open to negotiation over its role in life.

Remember the story from the last chapter about Oprah and the Jimmy Choos? She wore a size nine in every other pair of shoes she owned, but she knew she needed a different size in shoes by that particular designer. She could insist that she's a nine all day long, but until she kicked those Jimmy Choos off, she was going to be in pain. Pure and simple.

Of course, kicking off the bad fit is just the first step. If you don't find and connect with your true Self, you'll live out of alignment with your purpose and below your potential, winding up in one painful situation after another. Best case scenario, you end up like Jane with a series of caregivers who help you manage the pain in various ways.

If you really want to get somewhere—not just hobble around—you have to put on the shoes that fit. If you want to truly live—not simply survive—you have to align your daily actions with your authentic Self to be clear about your purpose and fulfilling your potential.

THE BEAUTIFUL EQUATION

When I told you how my life of suffering led me to discover and formulate The Method, I painted the picture in broad brush strokes, but I didn't get into the mundane details of how I ignored my Self on a daily basis. For example, I said I had an eating disorder, but what that really meant was that every time my body told me it needed food, I ignored that signal. I ate more than my physical hunger ever queued me to eat, trying to be "full-filled" through being full. I said I stayed in relationships with one man who mistreated me and another man who needed too much from me, but what I didn't explain was how every time I got pushed around or set up on a pedestal, I would intentionally silence the alarm bells in my head. I said that I worked my ass off for a company that I didn't believe in, but I didn't go into detail about how I would force my Self to express support for the very principles that struck me as phony.

My misalignments weren't limited to my diet, my relationships, and my job. I stayed up when I should have put myself to bed; I guzzled an extra cup of coffee when I should have taken a break from work; I went to parties when I should have enjoyed a quiet evening at home.

Just about everything I did on a day-to-day basis reinforced the cycle of doing the opposite of what my authentic

Self was calling for...and telling myself that it *was* what I really wanted.

By the time I discovered The Method, I realized I'd been betraying my Self since I was a child.

The only reason this epiphany didn't completely break me was because I simultaneously realized that everyone around me was doing the same thing. The truth was illuminated for me: we were all complicit in perpetuating a gigantic network of lies about who we were, doing things that were directly opposed to what our Selves were indicating they really needed in any given moment. This lifestyle of lying created stress and pain, which stole the potential of each moment as we lived it. Nevertheless, none of us was willing to do what should have been the obvious thing: tell the truth and break the cycle. No wonder most people can't answer the question about what their purpose is in life. It's impossible unless you actually live in integrity with your Self.

It wasn't hard to see why. One thing 99 percent of us share is an upbringing to judge our well-being based on external queues and feedback. This isn't surprising, given the primal roots of our social structure. The oldest part of the human brain is programmed to look at others for their evaluation of threats to the environment. In psychology, it's called social learning and it's what creates our Self-concept. It has its benefits, but when it's not remotely close to being balanced with a seriously connected relationship with ourselves, life feels incredibly conflicted and confusing.

Even though social learning goes as far back as mankind, we can all agree that humankind has evolved significantly since then. There are no prowling lions or roving packs of bandits on the horizon. Instead, our greatest threat these days comes from our closest relationships—a lack of expressed and actioned love effectively shared, a lack of communication, a lack of intelligent care.

Nevertheless, most of us are still living as though our well-being literally depends on other people's assessments. This starts from earliest childhood. Chances are good that when your parents told you to say please and thank you, to look both ways before crossing the street, to choose apples over cookies, and never to stick your finger in an electrical socket, they didn't say much about *why*.

Maybe they explained things to you in simple terms like, "It's better for you," or, "It helps you stay safe." Maybe they even gave you a short version of how calories or electrical currents work. But my guess is that you probably grew up the way I did—learning that safety (mostly social safety) and niceness were paramount, and that curiosity, experimentation, and nonconformity were less and less acceptable as you got older, and that's just the way life is. You just gotta keep your Self in check, or keep your shit together in a package that people are okay with...as if you could please everyone...it's crazy logic.

Imagine how different it would be if parents instructed their children like this: "I'm telling you this because it's a way that you can take care of your Self throughout your life and fulfill your amazing potential." Whether it was safety crossing the street or how to manage money or what to do when a boy wants to kiss you, what if they emphasized that everything they were telling you was a tool to be used by your internal navigation system in helping you live in integrity with your Self? What if your parents backed up that teaching by taking amazing care of themselves and fulfilling their own purpose and potential?

If that had happened, I'm willing to bet you wouldn't grow up seeing apples as the morally virtuous choice and cookies as the dangerous but oh-so-seductive enemy. There would be no good-versus-evil battle in your head between safety and indulgence, caution and comfort. Your internal navigation would be well practiced in making the best choice to fulfill your purpose and improve your potential.

As we grow older, our internal navigation starts to wake up. For some people, it happens as the whirl and tumble of their twenties gives way to greater stability in their thirties, and it suddenly dawns on them that their life has taken shape in a way they didn't intend. Others grind forward in grim confidence that things will get better once they reach the finish line of retirement. But then they realize when they get there that they've spent a lifetime ignoring themselves and losing their potential.

THE COMMON DENOMINATOR

One of the most rewarding experiences for me is seeing The Method work on patients who were considered "lost causes" by previous providers. In fact, the more a person's issues compound, the greater likelihood that their healing is right around the corner, provided they learn that connecting with themselves will put them on the practical path to living their purpose and potential. The most intense suffering is a sign of how hard the Self is straining against its constraints.

Often, those constraints are partly imposed by the patient's own loved ones. I've had to sit down for heart-to-heart talks with any number of devastated parents/ spouses/friends and explain that despite the vast amounts of wealth and resources they've put into helping their loved one, they have inadvertently played a significant role in creating the situation they are trying to fix.

The problem is that for these concerned family members, the patient isn't changing quickly enough or in the way the family expects. I have to point out to them that even though the patient is in a highly transformational process, they will continue to be impeded until they are set free from the pattern of trying to be the person their loved ones want them to be.

I tell them that I can help the patient completely reverse their downward spiral, that they can see their loved one happy, healthy, and thriving, but they will have to be ready for the pattern of their relationship to change. They will have to start getting to know their loved one's true Self, whoever that might turn out to be. While every single family member I've ever talked to says this makes more sense than anything they've ever heard, I can tell they are seriously scared of what this means—what they may have to finally face about their own relationship with themselves that they are afraid of. Although I know who the specific patient really is in the process, I take great joy in knowing that what I'm explaining, how I'm transforming their loved one's relationship with themselves, is communicating what the family member should be doing as well. It takes care of the family therapy part of things that almost all family members want to avoid doing at any cost...I just create a parallel process of guiding the patient and informing the family members so they can all begin to shift to a similar paradigm. They can create a healthy relationship with themselves, with integrity as the foundation.

The problem isn't that a patient's family and friends want bad things for them. It's that the patient's internal navigation is straining against the obligation to fulfill external expectations, and the resistance of an entire family system that is afraid of losing themselves. I get it. It's different, and it can be a radical shift to make, for some.

Most of us are taught from an early age that our parents know what is best for us—that our job is to simply follow their directions and respond to their correction. We're rarely taught to connect with our own Selves, let alone trust it over anyone else's direction. But the farther you stray from your true Self, the more you feel off track, and then the more inventive your Self will become in finding ways to show you that you are out of integrity.

OKAY...BUT WHY?

Whether it's Jane, or me, or you, we always come back to the big question: Why do we keep doing this?

Why do we keep overriding the signals from our internal navigation system?

Why don't we realign ourselves correctly as soon as we start to feel pain?

Why do we continue multiplying hurt upon hurt, lie upon lie, until we reach the point of crisis?

The answer is pretty simple.

We do it because no one around us ever told us there's another way.

Deep within the primitive, tribal brain lies the conviction that not only are each of us constantly in danger, but the key to our individual survival lies in supplying what those around us lack.

In modern-day terms, this translates to taking on other people's stress as our own and expecting others to serve us in kind by taking on our stress.

This is what motivated my family members to shift their pain onto me by confiding their worries to a seven-year-old child. It's what motivated me to shift my pain onto my parents by manifesting an eating disorder and then, when that backfired, to shift my pain onto two different husbands.

We absorb the pain and stress of others in the unconscious belief that they will do the same for us, and this is what most people refer to as "love." It's so instinctive that we don't even realize we're doing it. As a result, we usually don't realize that it's not working. This leaves most humans feeling burned in a fruitless transaction, instead of feeling love. Queue the need to look for "love" in all the wrong places, substances, and scenarios.

It's like that old "frog in hot water" metaphor, where the frog never jumps out of the pot because the heat is turned up one degree at a time until it's too late, and he's been boiled alive. We stay in painful situations without ever examining what the pain is telling us. We keep accepting the stress of others because we believe we need them to contain our own stress.

Meanwhile, everyone around us is confirming that stress is what we're *supposed* to experience. We're told that stress is just part of being a good employee, a good wife, a good daughter, a good friend.

What they really mean, whether they realize it or not, is that they are in pain and they expect you and everyone else to share that pain with them. After all, it's only fair.

Somehow, it never occurs to anyone that maybe we could all live without pain. Maybe if we stopped prioritizing this equal distribution of pain and each person focused on meeting their own needs by knowing their own hearts and minds, then more people could share the connection they have with themselves with each other instead of coming to everything from a place of lack and such need. This way people could connect to their own purpose and create their own experience of living their potential. Maybe then we'd start sharing something that made us all feel good and generated more of that feeling. It's being shared in a great synergistic way that generates a world of people living in their purpose and increasing the overall potential of our society. Think about how much we already produce with our brilliance, and what it would be like if we did this all through less Self-betrayal, more alignment with ourselves, and more enjoyment in general. Imagine what would change around us.

MAKING THE CONNECTIONS

I said before that The Method works because it starts with a commitment to your Self.

This is also the reason why The Method works *quickly*. Once you commit to learning about your Self, it doesn't take long to become utterly fascinated with your Self...

and rightfully so! Your regular check-ins will make you notice things you have never observed before—things you have felt your entire life and never once thought to inquire about.

You'll start to make the connections that your chronic migraines, acid reflux, or skin disease is directly tied to interactions that cause specific kinds of stress.

Then you'll start to connect those stressful interactions to more than just situations, but to deep-seated beliefs that you didn't even realize were running through your mind in those situations.

Then you'll examine where those beliefs came from, and you'll be able to make the distinctions between genuine internal conviction and external indoctrination.

That is the moment when, finally, you can let go of the misconceptions about yourself. As easily as releasing a balloon into the sky, the lies, misalignment, and pain float away; and often, so does the need for maladaptive coping mechanisms and medications that are about helping people tolerate a life that mostly feels intolerable.

The next stage is even better: once you've released what *isn't* your true Self, you start to dive into what *is*. You begin exploring what makes your body, mind, and spirit feel fabulous. You start to nourish yourself in every possible way, rather than feeling trapped in the push-pull of indulgence and deprivation. You feel less dependent on other people because you feel Self-ful. Perhaps most surprising of all, you'll find that the less you depend on other people to be something you need them to be, the more you genuinely enjoy them for who they really are.

If this sounds a lot like happiness to you, that's because it is.

Everybody's on a search for happiness in life, but the vast majority are seeking it from external sources. They never realize they're putting the cart before the horse— that until they have achieved happiness through a loving relationship with themselves, nothing else can possibly bring them true pleasure.

Happiness is not a goal to attain; it's a byproduct of living in integrity with your Self, knowing your unique life purpose, and being fulfilled through the experience of your full potential. As I said before, we don't have the option of living without obstacles, challenges, setbacks, and even tragedies. If we're honest, we don't even have the option of controlling our response to those things, because our true Self will always want to express what it feels. You can't nurture away your nature—your Self will always be there with you.

What you can do is invest a lifetime's worth of care into your relationship with your Self. Using The Method's tools of Self-inquiry and positive, constructive action will allow you to experience true happiness and fulfillment... not independent of your circumstances, but right in the midst of them.

If you've ever fantasized about a partner who would never let you feel alone...

If you've ever longed for a parent who always made you feel safe and protected...

If you've ever wished for a friend who would be your biggest fan and loudest champion...

That person is here, right now, inside of you. Isn't it time you made that connection?

Chapter Six

YOUR CHILD SELF AND YOUR ADULT SELF

———

Picture the cliché version of a psychiatrist. Seated behind a patient who reclines on a leather couch, he peers through tiny spectacles at the notepad in front of him, and then delivers that classic prompt:

"Tell me about your father."

It's a cliché because it's true. Despite the rapidly evolving landscape of different therapeutic approaches, they all have the common feature of dealing intensively with your relationship to the people who raised you.

It's a logical place for your relationship with your Self to start. After all, your relationship with a parent sets up the path for all your future relationships, whether the path you follow will feel practical or as off track as running into the same brick wall over and over. From an evolutionary standpoint, that paradigm-setting is much of the driving force behind parenting. They are there to take care of your basic needs, to protect and provide for you, so you'll grow into a healthy adult.

Where so many parents go wrong, however, is the direction they give you for all these life lessons. Rather than embodying well-being and Self-care, or even explaining how important those principles are as a practical roadmap for being the true Self you're meant to be, most parents focus on specific directions and corrections—*always do this, stay away from that*. Instead of helping you grow into a Self-sufficient adult, they're conditioning you to look outside yourself for the guidance and care you need.

No matter what life skills your parents may have taught you for functioning as an adult, odds are good that they sent you out into the world as an emotional child.

YOUR EMOTIONAL AGE

You should see the looks on some of my clients' faces

when I tell them that, emotionally speaking, they are somewhere between eight and sixteen years old. Most of them are shocked, even defensive. They'll remind me they've been running their company longer than I've been alive, or they'll tell me they received academic tenure when I was still applying for undergraduate admission. Some protest that they themselves have children who have wrung all the youthfulness out of them—they couldn't be immature if they tried.

I explain that I'm not discounting their knowledge, expertise, intelligence, or life experience. Far from it—I am fully convinced they have everything they need to construct a fulfilled and happy life. Yet, with all those resources, they're sitting in my sessions and going through my recovery programs, suffering from pain they haven't been able to control. Something has been limiting their freedom to live out their purpose and fulfill their potential.

This, I explain, is the very definition of an emotional child.

Adults are free, by law and by social agreement, to make their own decisions, act on their own initiative, and take care of their own needs. By contrast, children are quite limited in what they are free to do. They are dependent on others to feed them, clothe them, keep them safe, and generally make sense of the world for them.

Children often chafe against their limitations, but the upside is that they are typically absolved of an adult's responsibility for their decisions. That isn't the case for many people whose parents are complete disasters and they must become like adults from the get-go. A child may disobey their parent, flout their teacher's instruction, even commit a crime, and they will still be protected from much of the consequences that would attend an adult context for the same action.

No matter how well your parents raised you to manage adult responsibilities, it's very unlikely they spent equal time equipping you to manage or understand your emotions. Many families avoid emotions like the plague, which precludes any discussion of the Self or how to interpret communication from the internal navigation system.

That may not seem like such a big deal, until you consider how much of our practical functioning starts at the emotional level.

Even parents who diligently teach their children not to act on their destructive impulses spend very little time tying those impulses back to their root emotion. "Don't hit your sister" is good foundational training in impulse control, but it does nothing to help the child productively handle the emotion that provoked him to hit. Whatever

that emotion was—outrage, envy, desire for attention—
he'll be experiencing it again and again throughout his life.
Without knowing how to deal with this emotion, he won't
be connected to himself, which means he'll experience low
potential in general, and high potential for unintention-
ally Self-destructive or emotionally distancing behaviors.
Hitting his sister could later turn into hitting an enemy,
or hitting a girlfriend, or possibly even harming himself,
since what we do to others we typically do to ourselves
in many ways. Maybe that emotion won't manifest as
physical violence, but in some more insidious form of
harm—lying, cheating, addiction, isolation.

As you grow from childhood to adulthood, your muscles
strengthen, your brain cells multiply, and your spirit
expands. But your emotions are a different animal. As
ageless reflections of the true Self, they remain constant
throughout your life. Triggers may lose their power,
contexts may shift, but your anger will always be your
anger, your joy will be your joy, and your grief will be
your grief.

What can change, however, is your ability to recognize and respond to your emotions in a Self-connected,
Self-compassionate way that allows you to live more pur-
posefully, unlocking more potential in each moment. But
this only happens if you're given the tools to get started.

STOPPING THE MASQUERADE

If you're like most people in therapy, managing your emotions is your Achilles' heel, and you know it. No matter how busy your life is, no matter how hard it is to admit you need help, something within you feels volatile, impressionable, easily frightened, or ashamed.

This is why, in certain situations, you find yourself unable to control what you think, say, or do. You become unwilling to listen to reason, even when it's offered by people you trust. Despite your best intentions, you manifest a personality that makes you cringe in private, even as you deny it in public. You work hard to eliminate that trigger from your life, but you routinely find it cropping up whenever life feels too hard to deal with.

The context for these emotions, whatever it might be, isn't the problem. It's that deep down, you believe you are limited in your control *and* your responsibility regarding that emotion. Even when you're thoroughly ashamed of how you've behaved, something in you secretly feels you are not accountable for it, and that someone else is to blame for the harm you've caused.

You're hardly alone in this. The vast majority of adults out there are emotional children masquerading as productive members of society. The work of being a person hasn't been made practical to them; the mere idea feels too overwhelming to even bother trying. In this chapter, I'm going to show you how parenting, as it has been practiced for generations, conditions your Self to remain an emotional child, adding to your confusion as you chronologically age. I'm also going to show you how you can reverse-engineer your life to create an infrastructure for handling those emotions. This framework will help you mature every time an emotional conflict arises. Not only will your emotional Self quickly catch up to your chronological age, but your internal navigation system will even allow you to surpass it, revealing depths of wisdom that go far beyond your years.

I'll also tell you that developing emotional maturity is one of the most deeply rewarding parts of working through The Method. As your path unfolds before you, you experience a profound internal shift that gives you amazing access in being a person. The results of this shift are tangible. Don't be surprised if people start telling you that you look different. When your emotions are adult on the inside, it can't help but manifest on the outside.

I know it isn't easy to seek help, especially the kind that involves admitting a core immaturity. But look at it this way: by choosing to move forward in this process, you've taken the first step toward becoming an adult who lives each day in fulfillment of their purpose and potential.

"ADULTING" DEFINED

If you use social media, you've probably heard this newly minted word making the rounds: "adulting." It's a popular term with millennials, who use it to humorously describe the travails of transitioning from carefree childhood to grown-up responsibility. "Adulting" includes things like passing on a cute new pair of shoes so you can pay the utility bill, scheduling a dentist appointment before your social engagements, or doing your own taxes.

For people a generation or two ahead, it's easy to roll their eyes at this Self-congratulatory "adulting" phenomenon. Those of us raised before the millennials were a lot more prepared to meet the demands of adult life. The further back in history you go, the more true this becomes. Many of us have grandparents who, as soon as they hit puberty, were expected to work full-time jobs to support their family.

"Adulting," as popularly understood, means taking care of yourself. We can all agree it's pretty practical stuff, but do we really know the ultimate goal behind it? That is, who benefits from your ability to take care of yourself?

Answering this question will tell you a lot about your emotional maturity.

If I asked your parents, they would probably say you're the main person who benefits from what they taught you about taking care of yourself. But if I pressed them, and asked, "Why does your child need to know how to do that?" the benefit would probably stop being about you and start being about them. They don't want the burden of supporting a grown child, pure and simple. They did their work and they're ready for a rest.

By and large, parenting is commonly focused on directing and correcting—"Make sure to do this/keep far away from that"—with little (if any) emphasis on the *why* behind the mandates. People who were parented this way never learned to check in with themselves and align their actions with their true purpose and potential. As the years pass, this lack of alignment manifests as—you guessed it—an increasing level of pain.

Furthermore, when the parental relationship model is set up without clear alignment between purpose and action, it sets the paradigm for all future relationships to be out of integrity. If you're like most people, you've spent a good amount of your adult life trying to connect the dots between what you want from your relationships and how you always seem to end up behaving in them. Some people feel that misalignment so acutely that they make Self-sabotaging choices that end up hurting the very people they wanted to love. Think of a father who buckles under the pressure of raising his children and turns to alcoholism; a wife who feels she can't please her husband and exits the marriage; or an employee who pulls a "Jerry Maguire" and walks out on the job with no backup plan whatsoever.

The rationales these people give tend to be some variation on a single theme: "This isn't what I ever really wanted."

But even if that is true, exiting the situation is no guarantee of finding what they do want. In fact, statistics show us that people end up making the same relationship mistakes over and over again, just in new contexts. That's what I did in my marriages. I'm guessing you've done it in some form or another, as well. You may also notice the same themes or patterns taking place in all kinds of relationships—siblings, coworkers, neighbors, etc.

Our parents' effort to make us Self-sufficient backfired. Why? Because they never embodied real Self-connection. We absorbed the relationship that each of our parents had with themselves; the relationship they had with themselves taught us to be codependent in our future relationships with others. They weren't teaching us to be independent. Their approval-based dynamics for all of their relationships taught us to be even more codependent with more and more people.

It seems ridiculously simple when you really think about it. Shouldn't real Self-sufficiency focus on the sufficiency of your Self?

THE CAREGIVER'S ROLE

Think of the most dependent being that exists: the unborn baby. Cradled inside the mother's womb, it has absolutely no personal agency. It has no way of asserting its needs, wants, or will on the world. It utterly depends on the mother for its life, both in the present *and* in the future.

We're learning more every day about how nearly everything a mother does will affect how her baby is programmed and prepared for life outside the womb. No mother wants her baby to merely emerge from the birth canal alive and kicking. She wants it to come into the world with everything it needs to experience joy, success, and fulfillment. And because she knows she is the only one who can provide that for her baby, she has no hesitation in making demands on the baby's behalf. If she thinks that something she does could benefit the baby—taking an extra month off from work, consuming the highest-priced prenatal vitamins on the market, or enjoying a solitary spiritual retreat in the mountains—you'd better believe she's going to find a way to do it.

What's more, most people are going to *encourage* the mother to do these things. They may roll their eyes if she turns into "momzilla," but they recognize and respect the maternal mandate to go to any lengths on behalf of a baby's present and future health.

In fact, pregnancy may be the only context in which culture-at-large will step aside and let a person do what they believe they need to do, without judging her for being selfish or expecting her to have some consideration for everyone else.

Imagine that you had someone looking out for you this way in your life today. Imagine that you had a champion who did not give a hoot about what anyone else thought, but demanded that all your practical and emotional needs be met: that you get the physical and mental space you need, that you receive proper nourishment, and that your well-being must come before anyone else's.

I've got news for you: you are that person in your life. The practical path to your purpose and potential can only be experienced to the extent your relationship with your Self is one of real Self-sufficiency. This means you are the champion, protector, and caregiver for your Self, no matter what.

If it sounds outlandish, it's only because nobody ever modeled it for you.

ASKING WHY

When I sit down with my clients for our initial session, our focus is on their relationship with themselves. This practical roadmap to living their true purpose and potential definitely begins with talking about their parents. But we focus foundationally on how their parents treated themselves, and much more secondarily on the direct parent-child relationship dynamics. How did dad make decisions and what were the driving factors of his choices and behaviors? How did mom relate to herself and take care of her own needs? How did each of them talk to themselves, and how did the way they talked to you indicate what they felt about themselves and life itself? What was their set of core beliefs that motivated all they did or didn't do in their lives?

Most therapists would then ask the client, "How did you feel when they did that?"

Instead, I ask, "What does that tell you about your parent's relationship to himself/herself?"

Children are known to ask a lot of questions. They do this because they're trying to make connections between new information the world presents to them and the information they already have (or believe they have). What they never realize is that the adults in their lives are still trying to do that very same thing. Endeavoring to understand *why* is the throughline of living in the world.

In many cases, though, the child stops asking *why*. It may be because they reach a satisfying answer, but more likely, it's because the parent cut the conversation short with the classic response of the exhausted caregiver, "Because I said so," or, "It's just the way things are done."

Perhaps you remember how profoundly unsatisfying that answer felt in your "child" brain. There is no teaching in that answer—nothing to learn or inform you about being a person. This is why a person ends up feeling very impractical, stressful, and unfulfilled. You don't even have to be an extra sensitive or intelligent child for this to rankle; it feels as though your parent is concealing something from you. This breeds a feeling of insecurity.

But, in fact, this hyper-simplistic answer was entirely

truthful. Your parent grew up in a context where reasoning always led to a place where the buck stopped with somebody. It could be their boss, their religious leader, the president of the United States, or their very own parents. Somewhere in their life, there was a person saying, "You do this, because I said so." And when someone is providing the means for your very survival, then survival always trumps everything else. We accept what we think we must and carry that forward the rest of our lives, unless we awaken to a new reality.

In this context, there is no reference to the Selfhood of the person asking the question, outside of some token reference like, "Trust me, it's for your own good."

There is definitely no reference to the Selfhood of the person answering the question, "I tell you to do this because it benefits me in this way..."

Instead, every imperative is phrased as a universal. The less powerful ones are left to assume that the more powerful have a good reason to do as they've been told.

Do you see how that is the utter opposite of Self-sufficiency?

In the last chapter, I asked you to imagine a world in which a parent walked his children through the deep connections

of why they do what they do. But to do this successfully—
to avoid ending up at "because I said so"—the parent
would have to embody those same principles in their
own Self-sufficiency.

The child asks for a snack. The parent offers an apple. The
child asks why they can't have a cookie instead.

Most parents would say something like, "Because the
apple is good for you and the cookie is bad for you."

Maybe the parent would even go the extra mile and say,
"I'm giving you the apple because it's a healthy snack. I
want you to have a healthy snack, because I love you, and
I want you to be healthy. I want you to be able to make
healthy choices now so you can easily make those same
choices in the future and live the best life you possibly
can. Without your good health, there can be no real happiness, and without happiness, there can be no real health
and prosperity."

That's a perfectly decent interaction between a parent
and a child. But, let's roll it back a little farther—why did
the child ask for the cookie in the first place?

It's possible the child was simply testing the limits that the
parent had set for them. They know cookies are dessert

and they want to see if the parent will maintain order in their life.

But the most likely scenario is that they saw the parent, on numerous occasions, choose the cookie (maybe several of them) over the apple. To their child mind, focused on the present, it looks like the parent chose something deliciously sweet over something boring and ordinary—in other words, they chose pleasure over pain. So, when the parent says, "I'm giving you the healthy snack because I love you," all kinds of connections get made in the child's mind, such as:

- Health = boring
- Pleasurable = bad for you
- Love from my parent = deprivation of pleasure
- Being a grown-up = being able to choose what they say is bad for me over what they say is good for me

Whew! With a foundation like that, no wonder we're all so emotionally dysfunctional. Not only do we inherit a version of the world set in hyper simplistic terms—apples are good, cookies are bad—but every good and bad decision is attached to our parents' love for us and our love for them.

Henceforward, every time you choose apple over cookie, it's an expression that shows you are a good child, while every cookie chosen over apple is a resounding act of rebellion. As a result, you're thrown out of touch not only with what your internal navigation system really wants, but with the accurate context of "good" and "bad" for this scenario and all others.

Nobody tells new parents that their actions will literally imprint a "road map" in their child's psyche that he/she will follow as their path through life. Parenthood should be a moment where every person stops and thinks about whether what they are doing is working for them—whether their own relationship with themselves is designed to support them down the path that they want to go in life, a path that is not confusing and conflicting, a path that is designed to actually support them in loving themselves. Every parent has memorized the airplane rule, "Put on your own mask before you help your child with theirs," but they miss the deeper emotional equivalent of this rule. No parent can give their child the love they need if they don't first connect to themselves and live in integrity with their true Self and their needs. No parent can teach their child the life skills necessary to create a practical path to their purpose and potential without creating a practical path of their own.

The good news is that turning this around is a lot easier than you might think. You don't have to go back and fix your old decision-making framework piece by piece. Instead, you can scrap the old one and build a new one that is light, high-performing, and tailored to your exact needs.

STARTING FROM A PLACE OF LOVE

Taking care of your Self is indeed "adulting," but it starts with something much more fundamental than how you manage time and money, or even health and relationships. Being an adult means loving your Self enough to look out for its best interest in every situation.

It also means understanding that not every situation is made of the black-and-white, good-versus-bad broad strokes you learned as a child. The world doesn't work the way it does because someone out there said so. Rather, each of us works within the world and must assume the responsibility to live our purpose and potential in it.

The one universal we all have to interpret each situation, as it comes, is our internal navigation system. Without that grounding, we're forced to revert to the rudimentary system our parents gave us: this is good, this is bad. Whether we decide to be good rule-followers or bad little rebels, we're still making our decisions from the emotional age and capacity of a child. All our behavior is merely referencing past "Because I said so" moments, eliciting automated reactions that don't serve us, because each moment is new and requires a fresh perspective before proceeding.

By contrast, a mature person makes decisions from a deep wellspring of love for their true Self. This love is what lets them redefine pleasure as taking the best possible care of their Self, both in the present moment and in the future.

THE NEW FRAMEWORK IN ACTION

I recently attended a huge conference in San Jose for a well-known speaker. This conference had a carnival aspect to it; in between sessions, there was a big outdoor area with informational booths, people selling merchandise, and concession stands. This was a Self-improvement conference, so you'd think there would be some healthy, nourishing food there—but no, it was all nachos, pizza, and corndogs.

Even though I'm not normally attracted to that kind of food, after the rigorous session I'd just attended, it smelled pretty darn good to me. My friends and I were starving and, frankly, we didn't want to leave the festive atmosphere. So, we all ordered nachos; yes, me included.

But even as I was ordering my food, my internal navigation

system was working on my behalf. It knew that only a small part of me wanted the nachos, and not even the part that was hungry; it was more that I wanted to stay with my friends, to engage with the other people standing in line, and to soak up every moment of the experience we were there to share. My internal navigation also reminded me that I'd seen a Whole Foods Market in the strip mall a few miles up the road from the conference center; this meant I had the option of getting truly nourishing food at any point during our trip. Yes, I didn't want to miss a minute of the experience with my friends, and yes, the nachos rang those indulgent junk food bells, but my internal navigation knew that my true Self would be best served by taking a fifteen-minute break to go and get food that my body and mind actually wanted. Nourishing food, it told me, would provide the fuel I needed to fulfill my purpose and potential during that conference.

It's taking me longer to explain these thoughts than it actually took my internal navigation system to go through them. In reality, it was a split-second synapse that took place in the very act of choosing to eat nachos that afternoon. But once the day's final session was over, I took a quick detour on the way back to our hotel, stopped by Whole Foods, and stocked up on all my favorite real foods—yogurt, avocados, cashews, and some delicious quinoa salad from the deli. For the rest of the weekend, I had a healthy stash ready in my hotel room refrigerator, which allowed me to eat with my friends and still have the sustenance I needed to get the full benefit of the conference.

It didn't take long, it wasn't difficult, and I never thought twice about it afterward. At this stage in my life, my internal framework of loving my Self and following my internal navigation is so strong that those decisions happen pretty much on their own. After all, I've been practicing The Method for quite a while.

CHILD SEES COOKIE

When you first begin to implement The Method in your life, practical decisions like the one I just described will take a little longer. At this point, you may be in the habit of spending a lot of energy on small decisions like...well, whether or not to choose a cookie as a snack.

Maybe you didn't eat enough for lunch and an hour later, your body is pleading, "Feed me!"

Maybe you're low on energy and you're craving a sugar fix to keep you going.

Maybe you saw someone else eating a cookie and it made you want one.

Maybe you're having thoughts or feelings that you don't want to deal with, and your subconscious knows that a deliciously sweet cookie (with its vaulting sugar high and its subsequent crash and burn) will distract you for a while (another way your Self is trying to care for you).

Whatever the cause, there's a cookie on the horizon and you've noticed that some part of you "wants it."

It's easy to see the emotional child in this scenario. Kid wants cookie, kid goes after cookie. Maybe that's exactly what you do, and as you gobble down the cookie, you post-rationalize yourself as to all the reasons you deserved to eat it—post-rationalization being one of the hallmarks of the child-Self's strategy.

Or, maybe you get as far as the cookie jar, but then you stop. You think about how you're trying to cultivate a healthier diet. You reflect that you've already had enough sugar today; that's definitely what your mom would say, if she were here right now.

Just for fun, let's add a third voice to this conflict. Something else inside you says, "Mom is always nagging me about my weight. It's not like she's got that part of her life perfectly figured out, anyway. Why do I have to care what she'd think? I can do what I want."

This is a lot of conflict over a simple question like whether or not to have a cookie. It's really not supposed to be this hard to make a healthy decision about a snack.

Then again, this conflict isn't really about the cookie at all.

You already know perfectly well if the cookie is nutritious.

You also know whether the cookie contributes to you being able to thrive in your life (if you're trying to eat less sugar, if you're trying to fixate less on your weight, etc.).

What the cookie actually represents is your willingness and ability to take care of your Self. Here we are, back at "adulting."

ADULT SEES COOKIE

Now, let's talk about how an adult Self would handle this whole cookie scenario.

First, your internal navigation system is not the least bit shocked or scandalized to find that you want a cookie. Moreover, your internal navigation system doesn't attach any value judgment to that desire. It's not good or bad; it's merely present.

Your adult Self trusts your internal navigation system enough to lean into this present desire, examine the "why" behind it, and find the response that supports you in fulfilling your purpose and potential.

If you're physically hungry, you could take a few minutes to go out and purchase a snack that nourishes you.

If you need something to perk you up, you would be much better served by a twenty-minute nap or a walk through the park.

If you have been working hard all day and feel like you deserve a treat, then yes, you could eat the cookie. Alternatively, you could hold off until dinner, when you can order your favorite dessert and really take your time to enjoy it. Another option is that you could redefine "treat" as something that enhances your life beyond just something that tastes good in this present moment.

Your adult Self knows that what you do about the cookie right now isn't the main issue. It's the precedent you set for future situations—not just with cookies, but in all situations. If you choose to strengthen your adult Self in this cookie scenario, it's going to be that much stronger when you get a text from your ex, when your boss schedules you outside your availability, when your friend calls up with weekend plans she made without consulting you, and—yes, even this—when your mom calls to "check on you."

Your adult Self has the ability to decide whether any given desire is good for you—not good with a capital G, but good for you in the context where the desire shows up. Your internal navigation system is your ultimate caregiver. It gives you the power to stop simply reacting to external stimuli and to forge a reality where you are guided to make choices that support you in living out more of your potential in life.

That is the adulthood that your parents always wanted for you (and also for themselves). They just didn't know it, and neither did you, because we all live in a world of emotional children.

MOVING FORWARD

I said before that the emotional framework provided by The Method produces quick and tangible results. I should also warn you that the side effect can sometimes be intense embarrassment and even Self-chastisement for letting your "inner child" (as it were) run the show for so many years.

Let me counsel you not to spend too much time berating

your Self for this. Like I said, it's nothing to be ashamed of. You were given a very limited set of tools, and you were doing the best you could with them. And it doesn't help that your way of life was being reinforced by seeing childish behavior exemplified all around you from friends, coworkers, and culture at large.

We are all guilty of conditioning each other to be reactors to the present moment instead of being initiators of the future we truly want. The exciting thing is that, as you begin to develop into your emotional maturity, you could be the first domino that kicks off a renaissance of emotional maturity among everyone you know.

If that sounds grandiose, just think how your life might have changed earlier if you'd seen a good friend or family member modeling real emotional maturity by living out the kind of Self-advocacy that brings a sense of purpose and fulfilled potential in every moment. Remember, we always receive from the world what we put into it.

Honestly, though, the rewards of seeing your family and friends change is a distant second place to the reward of feeling your own emotional maturity begin to bloom. If asking the question *why* is the through line of living in the world, finding the answer within your Self is the source of endless fulfillment. Life becomes a journey of constant exploration, discovery, and wisdom. That's why the people who are going to evolve, regardless of circumstances, are the ones who commit to making practical choices that fulfill their purpose and potential.

Chapter Seven

TAKING AN INVENTORY

———

You probably came to this book the way my patients come to my office—heavy laden with a full list of issues that you want to fix.

I'll tell you the first thing I tell my patients, "Those issues are not your real problems. They are just the symptoms of the real problem."

Any therapist worth their salt knows that below the surface of any single issue, there is a lot more happening, maybe more than the patient is willing or able to acknowledge. That's why so many forms of therapy operate like a telescope—they start with one issue, then open out into bigger and bigger circles that encompass more of the patient's life, background, and psyche.

The Method works on the opposite principle. We start with getting as much on the table as possible, then scale backward so that we're only working with one specific aspect of a person's relationship with themselves and how that is playing itself out.

To many people, this feels completely counterintuitive at first.

"There's a lot of stuff I need to deal with," they tell me. Then they proceed to list the number of times they've bounced in and out of rehab, the years they've spent hiding sexual frustration from their unsuspecting spouse, their difficulty in showing love to their children. Some of them are even doing okay on the outside but, despite all their effort to conquer their demons, they still have a hard time feeling happy. Even when they are doing their best, they have this nagging suspicion that they are not living the life they are meant for. At this point, they're not sure that such a thing is even possible for them.

What they don't realize is that the whole time they've been listing their issues, I've been listening for something very specific. I don't see their issues as a set of discrete problems; I see them as the various loops and turns in one giant, snarled knot of unfulfilled potential. Knowing what caused the knot may offer some insight to this process, but to disentangle that knot, what I really need to find is a point of entry.

TAKING AN INVENTORY

To kick off my work with a patient, I have them create a comprehensive list of the fundamental impressions, beliefs, and patterns they have collected throughout their life, up to the present moment. What we're doing is taking an inventory of all their tools for solving problems in a world they cannot control.

Obviously, this list can get really big, really fast. That's why I have the patient focus on two main categories in creating this inventory: the beliefs that are rooted in parents and family, and the beliefs that have been developed through the actions of their daily life.

As soon as parents are mentioned, clients immediately think they know what's about to happen. They begin with lines they've rehearsed countless times in past therapy sessions, "My mother was never there for me," or, "My dad comes from a long line of alcoholics."

Naturally, your parents' choices have an impact on the

person you're enabled to become. The trouble is that most forms of therapy focus on the wrong set of choices.

As most of us understand it, the whole idea behind therapy is to fix troublesome behavior and mounting dissatisfaction with life by delving into its root causes. The hope is, by understanding where your parents were coming from, you can understand why they taught you the lessons they did. When a therapist asks you about your childhood, they're trying to uncover the foundational lessons you learned that now motivate you to do things you know are bad for you—overeat, choose the wrong relationships, skip your workouts, procrastinate at work, and so on.

But you can only work so far back in your own family history to find the root of certain lessons. How far back is far enough? At what point do you have enough information and enough understanding to finally break the pattern of your unproductive and Self-limiting behavior?

It's a terrible experience, no question, for a child to feel ignored by their mother or to witness their father's dependency on alcohol. But let's be real—you don't need a therapist to inform you that those behaviors were not good expressions of care toward you. Even if your therapist helps you develop compassion and forgiveness for your parents, years of awareness and understanding won't necessarily create major transformations in your default reactions.

Nobody's getting to the real *why* behind it all.

Except for The Method, that is.

INHERITING PAIN

Let's take the example of your father coming from a long line of drinkers. Odds are good that even when he was doing it, your father knew that he was repeating an unhealthy, destructive pattern. In fact, I'd be willing to bet that when your father was a young man, he swore he would never touch a drop because he never wanted to put his kids through the heartbreak he had experienced.

But as he got older and life started to get to him, that resolve began to break down. He started to resort to alcohol to take the edge off his personal pain, all the while reassuring himself that he wasn't the same as his father; he didn't yell, abuse, break things, hit his wife or children. What your father didn't realize was that the reason he was adding to the damage his father did, inflicting that damage on himself all over again, was because he had fully integrated the relationship his father had with himself and that was the core of the relationship he now had with himself.

The truly systemic issue wasn't what your father did when he was drunk; it wasn't even that he drank to deal with pain. It was that he accepted pain and allowed it to take a leading role in his life. He didn't know he could shift everything through creating an entirely different relationship with himself than his father had with himself. He didn't know he could make a shift in the present to be his own best friend and treat himself in a completely different way than his father treated himself. To be clear, neither of them knew this was an option, as most people don't.

Theoretically, your father could have been stronger. He could have summoned the fortitude to never drink at all. But that wouldn't have made him fundamentally different from his father. The truth is that if he hadn't been a drinker, the pain would have been channeled somewhere else—working too much, depression, ulcerative colitis.

The drinking was merely symptomatic of a much bigger problem—having chosen pain as a life paradigm. And because your father never dealt with it, this problem was always destined to be passed on to you in one form or another. If your father had had a good relationship with himself, instead of having absorbed the relationship that his father had with himself, he could have identified that pain and chosen to exchange it for a life of fulfilled potential. Once he did that, the drinking would have come into balance all on its own. More importantly, your father would not have passed on the burden of his default pattern of pain—the very problem that you find yourself dealing with now.

This burden can be passed on even if your parent is a stellar example. Maybe your father was loving and attentive, a dependable provider, a loyal spouse, present for all your sports games and music performances; nevertheless, you could feel the burden of his pain seeping through the cracks in his strength. Children are amazingly perceptive. Nothing gets past them, especially their parent's pain. The emotional energy that a child grows up under is more powerful than any loving or encouraging words ever said. Parents pass on the traits they embody, not the lessons they simply talk about or the directions they give.

I tell parents all the time that having a good relationship with themselves is the most important gift they can give their children of any age. Without it, children of all ages are destined to inherit stress, no matter how hard their parents work to be good moms and dads.

UNDERSTANDING LACK

Where does this inherited pain come from? It comes ultimately from the perception of lack—a systemic need for something you perceive you can't get on your own. Even more intensity comes with translating perceived lack in the present to painful lack in the future or, more simply, just pain in the future borne of not having the full potential of each moment.

We've talked a lot about perceived lack in this book so far—perceived lack of love, lack of knowledge, lack of care. But *lack* on its own isn't a word we tend to see. However, I use it this way because the whole point is that pain comes not from a specific, localized need, but from a general perception of insufficiency. In other words, you can have a very full life and be cognizant of your many blessings, yet still feel a chronic lack in your life.

Lack is that familiar feeling of "everything is great, but something's missing." It's what drives perfectly well-adjusted people to do crazy things like have affairs and get into credit card debt. It's what prolongs the cycle of addiction and abuse. It's what propels people to realize they are in the most fulfilling relationship of their life and immediately set to work sabotaging it. Perceived lack unites the wealthy with the indigent, the healthy with the ill, the spiritual with the atheist.

We talked in the last chapter about emotional maturity. Internal perception of lack is what creates emotional children. Just as actual children lack the financial, rational, and experiential resources to navigate the world on their own, emotional children lack—you guessed it—the emotional resources to navigate the world. They are constantly looking for someone else to protect them from their own feelings, guide them toward their purpose and potential, and supply them with the information they need to feel happy and safe.

To understand lack a little more, let's return to your hypothetical father.

He never knew that he had the option to take care of himself and heal his own suffering. Instead, he spent his life looking for someone else to take care of him—maybe your mother, maybe his workplace, maybe even you. The sad but true fact is that a lot of people choose to have children in the belief that those children will make them feel full and complete. They believe their lack will be filled by something of their very own to love, something innocent and untainted by the outside world. (It sounds a little creepy when you put it on paper, doesn't it?)

Unfortunately, when you parent out of perceived lack, you end up with an actual child being navigated through the world by an emotional child. Parenting from lack results in a child who is born into the job of filling someone else up. Needless to say, they are destined to fail at this impossible task, derailing their path to purpose and potential before they've ever had a chance to discover it. Instead, they are not in the business of trying to fulfill someone else's potential—an impossible task.

Your father did correct the symptomatic wrongs of his father—he doesn't abuse you when he's drunk. Maybe you'll do him one better—you'll grow up to be a moderate drinker, able to have a few beers and stop when you want. However, until you address the real *why* behind your pain and give your Self the loving attention it never received, you'll still be exactly like your ancestors were, experiencing life through the lens of suffering. However you choose to manage your pain, whether it's through socially acceptable means or some new level of outrageous rebellion, that core problem of lack will continue to plague your family lineage.

Had enough of this gloom and doom yet? I certainly have. So, let's move on to The Method and the power it gives you to break free from this cycle of suffering once and for all.

CULTIVATING AWARENESS THROUGH TAKING INVENTORY

The Method asks you to do an inventory with your Self on a regular and daily basis. This is a tool you'll be using constantly as you apply The Method. To do this inventory, you'll scan your body, mind, emotions, and spirit for places of pain, stress, confusion, or lack of direction. When you find one, you'll check in with your internal navigation system to find out what triggered those sensations.

You could do these inventories only on an as-needed basis, whenever conflict or pain grabs your attention. But I advise clients who really want to see transformation to start by doing their check-ins every fifteen minutes between the time they wake up and the time they go to bed. By doing it this frequently, you're accomplishing two things: You're heading off bad decisions at the pass by checking in with your Self before you subconsciously act out of perceived lack or pain (as opposed to waiting until you've made a whole day's worth of decisions that leave you in intense suffering). You're also developing a finely tuned radar within your Self. People who have ignored their own pain for years are often shocked once they start doing these check-ins, realizing how early their pain manifests internally—well before the pathological symptoms kick in. Your internal navigation system is very practical about signaling you about danger ahead, if you'd only pay attention to it.

By doing this inventory several times each day, you learn to be aware of your Self. This is a very different thing from what we understand as Self-awareness. Taking inventory has no reference to what other people think of you. Instead, it's all about checking in with what's going on inside you.

To see how the inventory works, let's create a fictional situation for you that will let us follow the whole process from start to finish. This chapter will be a little longer than the others, but I promise that seeing how the inventory process plays out in this scenario will help you understand how to apply it to your Self.

DOING THE INVENTORY

Your alarm wakes you up at 6:00 a.m. You take a moment to check in with your Self and find that you're feeling grumpy.

When you ask yourself why you're grumpy, you could respond the easy way: "I hate my life" is a reliable classic. Or, you could reach into the memory vault for something like, "Getting up early takes me back to high school, which I hated."

But remember our rule against false narratives? If we stick only to verifiably accurate Self-talk, taking inventory can start transforming your bad feeling into powerful action on behalf of connecting to your purpose and living your potential.

Is your bad mood stemming mainly from physical discomfort? Maybe you didn't get enough rest or maybe you're starting to get sick.

Is it mainly mental or emotional? Maybe you're dreading your commute. Maybe you had a conflict with someone yesterday and it's still bothering you.

Is there anything about your feelings regarding your job in the mix? It doesn't have to be about your job as a whole; maybe it's just something about today that is getting you down. Maybe you hurt your back over the weekend and you're afraid of spending all day sitting in your office chair. Maybe you have a presentation due, but you're anxious about talking in front of people. Maybe you ate poorly the night before or are dehydrated. Whatever the reason, your Self is signaling you to investigate.

Each inventory session offers you a little more information about how your Self is responding to the input of the world. It turns your whole day into a scavenger hunt where the clues about how to live your purpose and potential get revealed to you, one fifteen-minute session at a time.

Each time you practice it, the inventory process shows you a little more of your Self, giving practical insight you can use to create your unique path.

After about two weeks of these consistent check-ins, something amazing happens: you become an expert on your Self. It may sound incredible, but it really only takes that short amount of time to get in sync with your internal navigation system. Once you really make an effort to listen to what your Self is telling you, your Self rewards you with plenty of information. (I told you that all it wanted was your attention!)

You'll also find that because your Self is assured that you are paying attention, your symptoms of pain start to lessen. The stomachaches aren't as sharp; the moods aren't as intense. As you continue to do your inventories, the process quickly becomes less regimented and more intuitive. You find yourself doing inventories without having to set a timer or even think with the same level of deliberate intent. Instead, there's an increasingly seamless flow between sensation and reflection. You're getting in tune with your internal navigation system, and you're putting the pieces together of your perfect path for your life and it becomes incredibly practical. Your life is finally starting to feel easy and natural, the way it was always meant to be.

The first two weeks are really just about collecting information and observing patterns. Once you've got a healthy file of evidence to work from, that's when The Method—your Method—goes into healing overdrive.

Now, when you do your inventory, you not only check in with your symptoms, but you probe a little deeper into your Self. With each symptom of pain that you note, you ask your Self the following questions:

QUESTION 1: "WHAT WERE MY INTENTIONS DURING THIS TIME?"

Remember that intentions are not the same as goals. In asking this question, you're not trying to get at the material outcome of your actions, but at the internal desire that drove you to take that action.

You can take it a little deeper and ask where those internal desires come from. Are they genuinely your desires or were they taught to you by someone else? If so, does your true Self resonate with those desires or is your true Self drawing you toward something that will feel more purposeful and fulfilling?

QUESTION 2: "WHAT OBSTACLES CAME UP WHEN I TRIED TO REALIZE MY INTENTION AND FAILED?"

Even if your action leads to a successful material result,

it may not yield a corresponding success within your Self. For example, you may spend your whole workday with a stomachache stemming from your anxiety, even after your presentation is over.

QUESTION 3: "WHERE DID I REALIZE MY INTENTIONS WITH FEW OR NO OBSTACLES?"

This is the other side of the coin. Sometimes your intention does lead to a great internal feeling of success, even if the outward signs are less than stellar. Maybe your stomachache disappeared during a few moments of your presentation, and you really sensed how your actualized potential was contributing to the success of your company. Explore that and ask your Self what it was experiencing in those moments.

QUESTION 4: "WHAT FEELS PARTICULARLY RELEVANT TO YOU?"

Every situation provides a lot of information; often, it provides more than is truly helpful. As you take inventory in each given situation, it's important to stay away from navel gazing. (Keep in mind that you'll have another opportunity to check in with your Self in just fifteen minutes.) There's no need to push too hard for the relevant pieces to appear. Just ask your Self and it will volunteer the information you need.

QUESTION 5: "WHAT PATTERNS DO YOU OBSERVE?"

Sometimes patterns are obvious right away: *I get anxious when I speak in front of people, and my anxiety goes straight to my stomach.* But try asking your Self for insight that goes a little deeper and you may be surprised by what emerges.

Is there someone whose pleasure you visualize when you do things that are out of integrity with your Self?

When you do something that isn't aligned with your true purpose, do you feel you achieved less potential and then "buy" your Self's permission by promising your Self a "reward"—especially one that doesn't contribute to your living closer to your purpose and potential?

How do you respond to other people for the rest of the day after doing something out of integrity with your Self?

What do you find your Self thinking about as the day goes on? Are those thoughts and ideas positive/productive or negative/destructive to your Self, or are they more purposeful and taking you down the path toward more potential?

FINDING THE ENTRY POINTS

You might have noticed that there are multiple points of entry into this whole inventory process.

There's how you feel physically—fatigue, muscle tension, immune system breakdowns, skin issues.

There's your emotional state—anxious, lethargic, irritable, melancholy.

There's your mental condition—hyperaware and over-stimulated, or else drifting in a brain fog.

Your instinctive actions, or should we say reactions, are another point of entry. This includes things such as whom you choose to call, which addictions start calling your name, how you treat your responsibilities, and whether your behavior becomes destructive or constructive.

Finally, and perhaps most important of all, there is the point of entry provided by your Self-talk. Self-talk is a particularly key point of entry because it usually precedes the other responses. In other words, the narrative you are imposing on your Self is what provokes your Self to start signaling for help in the form of pain or behavior.

EXAMINING THE NARRATIVE

Typically, it can take a few weeks to a month of inventory sessions before you're able to tune into your internal narrative in a more automated way. But once you start to perceive it, you'll rarely miss it again. Examining the narrative is the crucial component that allows you to complete The Method's final element: acting on what you know to be true.

If you're like a lot of people, you spend a lot of time on narratives filled with impractical language, particularly the words, "I have to." As we've already seen in Chapter 4, words like "have to" or "should" or "can't" are nearly always signals that the narrative is false.

Just for fun, let's take an example narrative: "I have to do a good job on this presentation," and let's pick it apart.

I used to fall victim to this same statement a lot, until I used The Method to dig deeper and inquire what would actually happen if I didn't get the work done. Somebody might get annoyed or maybe feel let down. Possibly, the progress of some project would be delayed. The real question became whether those possibilities were worth stressing my Self out over, time after time. When it became a contest between someone else's convenience and my personal well-being, did I deserve to lose every single time?

Let's shift it back to you and the fictional presentation you "have to" do. What is the worst-case scenario if you *didn't* do a good job? That you'll get demoted or fired from your job? We're working off the assumption that you are a hard worker and have been reliable and consistent in the past. Given your track record, is it likely that you'll get fired for doing a just-okay job this time?

If the worst-case scenario did happen and you did get fired from your job, the presentation would still get done, because somebody else would be given the task in your absence. You can't be the only person with the expertise to get this presentation finished. That means you probably have the option of seeking support to get it done. You could even make that the action you take on what you know to be true.

For now, though, let's realize that this is not a "sky is falling" situation. This is a situation in which you have options. The words "have to" don't belong in this situation at all. They are a completely false narrative that serves no purpose, other than to get in the way of following your internal navigation to fulfill your purpose and live your full potential in this moment.

A DEEPER REALITY

It's now time to delve deeper into acting on what you know to be true, which means it's time to talk about the matrix.

Forget anything you might be thinking about freeze-frame flying or red pills versus blue pills. This matrix is a lot more visceral than the sci-fi movie version. It does, however, deal with discarding perceptions and working within a deeper reality.

Matrix simply means "a surrounding medium or structure," and The Method asks you to start approaching your life within the surrounding medium of your Selfhood.

As you do your check-ins and take inventory, you'll start seeing patterns for how you deal with various situations and contexts. You'll see that in certain settings, you're able to act in accordance with your intentions extremely well. These are the situations where you actualize your unique potential, allowing you to live out that situation in integrity with your Self.

In other settings, the opposite will be true. You'll have a hard time following through with your intentions. You'll live out the situation feeling frustrated and unfulfilled because your potential was left untapped.

You'll start to notice not only where these strengths and weaknesses manifest, but whether there's a tie-in amongst them. Remember my story in Chapter 3—I was able to follow my internal navigation extremely well in my career; but in my romantic life, I was a lot less in integrity with my Self.

Taking note of these patterns is merely in service of creating your matrix, which means it should be done completely without judgment. As you start to see the medium in which you exist as being made up of areas where you are more or less in integrity with your Self, you'll be able to develop the ability to apply the strength in one given scenario to the scenario where you are in less alignment with yourself.

Remember how I shared the epiphany I experienced in my earlier career? I realized that I was telling lies for a living, which made it no wonder that I was getting back lies in return. The choice to pursue more integrity and honesty in my work affected not only my professional life, but my romantic life as well.

When I work with clients, they may have ten or twenty or a hundred issues that need to be addressed. It's overwhelming to develop and adopt new practices for every area of your life all at once. That's why we focus on one aspect of their life at a time. By starting to change just one aspect of your life, you learn to work with the fundamental tools that create change. It creates a "muscle memory" deep in your psyche. The more effort you put into making this shift in this one area of your life, the more you experience its efficacy in connecting you with your purpose and potential, which naturally motivates you to implement it into other areas of your life. Before long, connecting to your purpose and living your potential becomes just as automatic as the previous pattern used to be. You start to experience the rewards of living in integrity with your Self in one area, and your mind, body, and spirit instinctively want to create that same integrity in all areas of your life.

When I started being more truthful in my work, I organically gained the ability to be more truthful in my dating life. I didn't have to be the perfect version of whatever woman my date wanted—I had the freedom to be my Self, open and honest.

This change also affected the way I treated my body. As I progressed in honesty toward others in various contexts, I was increasingly able to be honest with my Self about what was best for me to eat, how I wanted to exercise, and how much sleep I needed at night. My body relaxed and flourished under this care. Within just a few months,

I went from feeling comfortable in my own skin to feeling truly amazing.

Let's add the matrix into the fictional example we've been using, and see what happens.

BUILDING THE MATRIX

You made a decision that you weren't going to abide by the false narrative of "I have to do a good job on this presentation." Instead, you chose to be honest with your Self and proactive in seeking help. As a result, you did a better-than-average job on the presentation, and you got a pat on the back from your supervisor afterward.

Normally, you'd just take the commendation and move on with your day. However, today you are armed with a lot of great information from your inventory-taking session. This gives you a unique opportunity to take action by articulating your truth.

"I'm glad you liked it. It actually went way better than I expected because I was able to get help from a coworker. I think in the future it would be helpful for us to team up on presentations like this, so we can all get the best possible value for our time in the meeting."

I mean, damn. What supervisor wouldn't respect that?

Congratulations—this part of your professional life has officially become an area of strength in your matrix. Now, let's apply that same strength to an area of weakness. Let's make it about another "should/have to" scenario: "I really should call my mom regularly."

You know your mom lives for your calls so she can "check in" on you. She asks a lot of questions about what you're eating, if you're dating the right people, when you last visited the dentist, or got your oil changed. You know, all those mom questions that really shouldn't be asked of someone your age.

You want your mom to know you love her, so you keep calling her and letting her do her thing. But today, things are different. You've just come off a very powerful turning point of not letting past patterns dictate future behavior. Instead, you apply the strength that helped you be honest with your supervisor to being honest with your mom. This could look one of two ways.

The first way is that you choose not to call your mom. You know you love her and, if she chooses to be honest with her Self, she would know it, too. But you see that her compulsive admonishment of you is really symptomatic of her not having a good relationship with her Self. You can't fix that for her, and pacifying her through regular calls isn't ultimately serving her purpose and potential or your own.

The second way is that you do give her a call. But when the questions start, you say something like this: "Mom, I love you and I'm really glad you care about me. I had a great day at work today and I'm doing really well. I've only got a few minutes to talk, so I'd really like to hear how *your* day went."

Imagine what life would be like if there were no such thing as "have to." That's what integrity means—all the options are up to you. Just a day without doing anything out of obligation could be all you need to experience the truth—that nobody dies if you do only the things that come naturally, easily, and freely. You're still breathing at the end of the day. The world is still turning. Your loved ones are just as safe as they were before. There really is no such thing as "have to."

In Chapters 8 and 9, we'll get into more of the potential outcomes of shifting these patterns. But for now, ask yourself what's so wrong about doing something different from the way you always do it. You know what life is like under the false narrative. If your purpose and potential are not being fulfilled by the way you're doing things now, isn't it time you tried something new?

TOO MUCH OF A GOOD THING

We all know how common it is to dive into one pursuit that makes us feel super successful, because we need to compensate for the parts of our life that feel unsatisfying, debilitating, or fraught with pain. As you work on building your matrix, you'll also start seeing where your areas of strength may actually be making you weaker in other areas of your life.

Think back to my personal story for a moment. I shared that I was drawn to my abusive boyfriend because his way of making me feel lovable, accomplished, and awesome made up for the way I felt I never measured up to my family's emphasis on physical attractiveness and success. Later, of course, that part of my life started to get weaker, so I threw myself into my professional career.

When you do this, it winds up working against you. By using an area of strength to deflect your attention from areas of weakness, you actually trap your energy and power in a specific part of your matrix. Trapped energy rebounds on itself and becomes addictive, compulsive, unstable. What happens then is your areas of strength actually hold you back from growing.

Think of it this way: carrots are good for you, but if you only ever eat carrots, you're going to have a nutritional imbalance. Sleep is good for you, strength training is good for you, sex is good for you, but you need to find the right amounts of all these things that are appropriate for your individual Self.

This is where we come back to where we started—parenting your Self. You have the responsibility to identify areas of development in your matrix and systematically apply The Method, which gets easier and easier the more you apply it in your areas of strength.

By doing this, you do more than simply supply balance to your life. You systematically eliminate lack of full potential from your internal landscape. You never have to refer your problems back to your parents' issues or anyone else's, for that matter. Instead, you experience the transformative truth that you are all you need to live your purpose and potential. You have everything you need to take care of your Self, and the more you do it, the more your Self will take care of you.

Chapter Eight

BECOMING YOUR OWN CONTAINER

Our brains have an amazing ability to unconsciously imitate or adopt whatever behavior we are exposed to. This is the result of particles known as "mirror neurons," and they are the reason why, among other things, children learn from what their parents do rather than what they say.

Mirror neurons are also behind The Method working so quickly for patients. When they meet with me, they finally get a chance to see someone model living in integrity with themselves. While they may not see me eating nutritious food, practicing ballroom dance, or interacting with my friends and family members, they feel the effect of all those tiny choices in the way I treat them. They feel, often for the first time, what it's like to have someone care for them without the burden of expectations. They experience what it's like to be instructed without the feeling of being judged or needing to meet my needs because I failed to tend to my own Self.

The small choices I make to live in integrity with my Self yield a hundredfold when the client, seeing true health for what might be the first time, is provoked by their own neurotransmitters to emulate what I'm doing. Without realizing it, they pick up my turns of speech, my posture, my attitude toward life, and they run with it, adapting it to serve their own purpose and potential. One of my favorite parts of coaching is the way my patients teach me what they discover as they connect with themselves on such an intimate level and experience their potential for what might be the first time in their life. I'm inspired all over again when I witness their sense of wonder (and relief) that they have finally found their practical path... and it wasn't even that hard!

This is just more proof of how much your true Self wants to be cared for. Your Self's desire to be nurtured is so great that when it sees someone else loving and caring for themselves, it will create intense cravings in you to be around that person more often. Your Self wants to live in that environment of nurture, even if it is simply emanating from someone else.

However, I'm clear with patients that The Method doesn't let you settle for transferring your relational dependency onto one person who helps you contain your feelings. Instead, real healing begins when you can build off that person's own Self-containment to begin containing your Self.

YOU ARE YOUR OWN SAFE SPACE

While it doesn't take many weeks of internal check-ins to realize your power of fully taking care of your Self, it also doesn't happen overnight. The process of realizing your weaknesses and probing into your intentions can be a little exhausting, especially on an emotional level. Your initial forays into taking care of your Self and making better choices may be halting and clumsy, like a child learning to walk. It's normal to feel sudden, intense fears that the world may come crashing in, followed by a "withdrawal" experience as that fear exposes a little more of how others-dependent your sense of Self has been.

As a coach, my job is to serve as a temporary safe space. I help your Self relearn the feeling of experiencing emotions in safe containment. In helping you course-correct when needed and offering direction, I serve as the proxy for your true Self as it detaches from needing care from all other sources in your world.

What really makes the difference in this model is that I'm serving as that proxy within the boundaries set by my own relationship to my Self. In other words, I'm not "there" for patients to the same degree that I am there for my Self. In learning to trust me, they are learning they can also trust me to take care of my Self first and foremost. Their brain subconsciously registers the message that this is the behavior they must adopt if they are going to live in integrity.

PUTTING YOUR SELF FIRST

Most of your life, you have seen everyone you love putting someone else's well-being before their own. Your parents may have put yours before theirs, or they may have put your sibling before yours. Maybe your spouse used to put you first, and then they started putting their aging parents or their work before you.

Why do people do this? Again, it's because we don't know any other way. We are habituated to throw ourselves into whatever relationship we think will compensate for our perceived lack of Self. And in the event that we're left without anybody who gives the illusion of compensating for that lack, that's when we fall headfirst into our addictions.

We subconsciously expect and demand that other people

in our lives contain us because we believe—again, subconsciously—that we cannot contain ourselves. The perversed truth of it all is that the only way any one person can serve adequately as a container for someone else is when they have grown adept at being their own container.

Having practiced The Method as long as I have, I know what it takes to make this transition. It was only after several of my loved ones—my father, my mother, my grandmother, my husbands—proved unable to protect me that I finally decided I could not rely on any of them to contain my pain, much less provide an example of how I could contain it alone.

I still wasn't ready to trust my Self fully, so I found a container in the teachings of the people I mentioned in Chapter 4. Fortunately, my internal navigation system alerted me to the fact that each teacher that helped me had drawn from the wisdom of someone else. Instead of one teacher becoming my sole container, I was intuitively prompted to assemble all the teachings I discovered into a framework for containing my Self.

In a very real way, serving as your own container is the same as reparenting your Self. In giving you these tools, I'm doing for you what your parents would have done if they'd known how. Lucky for you, reparenting your Self through The Method doesn't take eighteen years. You don't have to "reenter the womb," rehash old stories, or seek apologies from the people who have harmed you. All you need is a new example to pattern your Self after, and a safe space where your volatile emotions can be safely contained as your metamorphosis takes place.

In my experience, the Self doesn't need more than a year or two of this consistent work to relearn a healthy Self-care system. It will amaze you how quickly the new patterns begin to set in as you practice them.

HOW THE PRACTICAL PATH WORKS

A member of my team used to work in a role known as a "sober companion" to people who had just come out of rehab. His whole job consisted of monitoring people who had completed their program but were too fragile to deal with life at the most basic level. These were people for whom the smallest conflict or challenge would send them running back to the liquor store or to their opiate supplier. My colleague's job was to be present with a patient around the clock and available for support in every conceivable situation. He'd accompany the patient to the DMV to get their driver's license back. He'd help them shop for groceries. He'd do their dishes and even scrub out their toilet. If they wanted to talk, he'd listen. If a phone call made them upset and agitated, he would take the phone and end the conversation on their behalf.

Being the patient's long-term companion isn't a long-term solution. Rather, his job was to help the patient acclimate to normal life again. Their lives had revolved around their addiction for so long that they had lost touch with how to overcome the smallest obstacles. They needed to learn how good it felt to function as an emotional adult: living in a clean house, eating nutritious food, having healthy friendships. He was there to accompany them as they moved through the effort of taking care of themselves in daily life, without buckling under the stress and resorting once again to Self-medicating. He was there to assure the patient of their own Self-efficacy until it became so natural to their body and mind that they could carry on without him.

Being a container is a lot like that. While my team and I don't personally live with our patients, we help them relearn the basics of taking care of themselves, affirm their good choices, and help them learn from the choices that were not so good. I/we set them up in a new pattern of living by providing feedback until their own body and mind begin to develop a productive feedback loop of their own.

At its most basic, the container process means providing

accurate information about any given choice, whether it manifests in thought or in actions. If a patient says to me, "I'm having lunch with my dad later and I just know it's going to make me want to stick my finger down my throat and throw up," I respond by saying, "Okay, that's a choice you can make. But first I want you to connect to your Self and ask how you will justify that choice. What can you tell your Self that would justify why you want to hurt it? What is your real purpose in this life and how would that choice impact the potential of your quality of life in the present and set up a negative pattern for the future?"

This is an entirely new way of thinking for most patients. They are lost in a negative feedback loop of pain, Self-medication, and punishment. Even though they want to change, the only way they know to motivate themselves is through negative reinforcement, using the exact same behaviors that caused them harm in the first place.

My job as a container is to help them acclimate to the idea of making Self-advocating, productive choices that express love and care for themselves right now, which is where all of life's potential lies. Even in the process of making those choices, they may be emotionally volatile, fearful, and susceptible to triggers. As their coach, I serve to contain them through that process, assuring them they are creating a pathway that their nervous system will adopt over time, that what feels so wrong and unsafe to them is actually helping them create a new default "setting" that will make it easy to move out of struggle and into a life of purpose and potential.

As the work progresses, the patient moves from being contained to containment. They begin to shed the external container as they become stronger and begin to contain themselves. In the same way that a butterfly breaks out of its chrysalis, unfolds its wings, and stretches them for flight, the client looks less and less to their coach for reassurance and begins to reassure themselves, without prompting or guidance. The client is becoming their own coach. It's a beautiful thing to see happen.

What makes this possible is when the client has fully internalized The Method. The process of check-ins is happening automatically, at a level beyond thought. Like the example I gave of choosing healthy food over three days of nachos at the conference I attended, you become able to follow the direction of your own internal navigation system with little to no interference from past patterns. What used to manifest as pain is barely a blip on the radar—your true Self is able to course-correct with the smoothness and sensitivity of power steering on a Porsche.

When you begin living in integrity with your Self in each

practical choice you make, you are truly living out the path of your true purpose and full potential.

BEYOND NORMAL

If you're like a lot of my clients, you have this idea that normal life is unavailable to you. Your weight balloons when you eat what your friends eat; you go off the rails when you have just one drink; you sabotage yourself every time a new love or a new career opportunity shows up. You've stopped hoping for an amazing, fulfilling life and your highest aspiration is just to be average.

Maybe at this point in your journey, The Method just feels like another medication to help you manage your pain and make up for your deficiencies. You hope it will work, but using it feels like more proof that normal life will never be available to you.

I'll grant you that life under The Method is nothing like the "normal" you're used to—a hot mess of stress, sickness, and dissatisfaction. It's the kind of abnormal that unusually beautiful or wealthy people experience, or rock stars or sports celebrities or geniuses. You're a normal person, but you're living life on a different plane from most, and people can't help but be in awe of it.

Depending on the severity of your issues, you probably expected that following The Method for the rest of your life would be like taking a medication or adhering to a strict diet—a regimented lifestyle that continues to single you out from other people, serving as a dead giveaway that you can't be like everyone else and just live life.

In fact, nothing could be further from the truth. Far from chaining you down to a lifestyle, a routine, or a schedule, The Method sets you free to live life however you choose. The more you assimilate the patterns of checking in, using accurate and affirmative Self-talk, and applying the strengths of your matrix to the weaker areas, the more you will be master of your own emotions, your own body, your own mind. There are no more regrets, no more mistakes—just an ever-unfolding path leading from one interesting, fulfilling, awe-inspiring experience to the next. You'll begin to feel like you're walking around with the secret to life in your back pocket...because you are.

It's impossible to overstate the feeling of having your life truly feel like your own. The whole push-pull of Self-control fades into the background because you can hear what your Self is actually asking you for. Remember, as we said back in Chapter 6, it always asks you for what is best. The language of "rewarding yourself" will become meaningless to you, as will "punishing yourself." Because you are actively loving your Self and connecting with your purpose and potential in each moment, you won't be locked in a pain/control struggle anymore. You will be free.

LIVING IN A MYSTERY

One of the hallmarks of life, no matter where or how you live it, is its constant uncertainty. For many patients, this is the ultimate layer of pain and suffering—they feel good now, but what will happen tomorrow, next week, ten years from now? This is often where people regress just as they show signs of real progress. They fall in love with someone really good for them, and then they freak out because they feel uncertain about what marriage will mean for them. They stop bingeing and move out of their parents' home, then feel uncertain about their ability to manage food when it's not the currency of their relationship.

But once you've practiced putting your Self first, you feel a settledness, even in the moments where you don't know what's coming next. Uncertainty and doubt are transformed into wonder and interest. You know that your Self will respond to every situation with a frank, honest presentation of what it needs in that situation, and your Self knows you can be trusted to give it what it needs. There's nothing to be afraid of in that situation, is there? Just like a child can go anywhere in the world if they are holding their parent's hand, you will have every confidence that you can give your Self whatever it needs, without any need for pain or struggle to get your attention.

I like to tell clients, "There isn't a problem I can't help you solve, even though I don't live in a problem paradigm." This makes them scratch their heads at first, but by the time they have mastered the art of containment, they nod knowingly when they hear it.

The only real problem you'll ever have is not being able (or refusing) to hear your Self articulate its needs to you. Outside of that, every situation is just a situation. You don't need to be able to predict your environment because there isn't anything that can hurt you beyond your ability to heal your Self. Your practical path is most evident when you choose to advocate for your own Self and its potential, especially in moments of challenge and difficulty. In fact, you may experience greater potential in those difficult moments than other people do in an entire lifetime.

Chapter Nine

DOING IT FOR YOUR SELF

———

You know the saying: "More money, more problems."

I can tell you from personal experience that this saying hits the mark. The world offers you plenty of distractions from dealing with your issues and, when money is no object, the more easily and inventively you can use those distractions—as well as the priority of making more money—to deflect the signals from your internal navigation system.

These days, my team and I spend the bulk of our clinical hours with fantastically wealthy people who have gotten themselves into fantastically complicated scenarios. By the time these people show up in our programs, they are completely spent. Their spirit, their intellect, and their physical bodies are exhausted with the intensity of their struggle.

It's my privilege to help them, but it takes a lot of effort and dedication, not only to our programs and in our sessions but also in cross-referencing their issues so we can connect them with supplementary forms of therapy. Nutrition, hormone replacement, drug rehabilitation, naturopathic remedies, genetic and neuropsychological testing, extensive lab work, sometimes even major surgery—all of these play a part in restoring a person to function in service of their true Self.

However, these patients tend to be people who—how shall I say this?—haven't had to do things for themselves the way most people have. Many of them have spent most of their adult life surrounded by various kinds of support staff—assistants, nannies, agents, entourages. As a result, they might not have ever had to develop into adult levels of responsibility for daily life, much less for their internal well-being. To put it bluntly, some of these folks need more intensive support until the emotional maturity piece kicks in.

When that happens, they suddenly see their relationships with startling new clarity. They can let go of what isn't needed. They can be selective about how much they engage. They can form relationships on the basis of what feels intuitive, instead of out of dependency.

We've talked about a lot of ways The Method is different from other forms of therapy. It works amazingly quickly; it focuses on progress instead of on the past; it detaches you from dependency on others. Another big difference is that The Method's goal is to get you out of therapy. All our coaches are trained in empowering you to create your own practical path through the power of the relationship with your Self.

Remember, nobody taught me The Method—I assimilated it through an array of different teachings filtered through my internal navigation system. Even as you're learning to implement what this book has taught you, your navigation will be showing you ways to adjust, shift, and customize these tools for greater precision in your own life.

And that's exactly how it should be. I can't say this enough: The Method is really no more complicated than simply listening to your Self, acting on that information, and allowing that process to deliver what you've been longing for, which is a sense of purpose and the fulfillment of your potential.

You've already taken the first step in this new lifestyle by reading this book. Congratulations—you're connecting to a practical path toward the effortlessness of being you! But maybe being this close to the final chapter has you feeling anxious, wondering what happens when the book is over.

No need to worry. The Method is set up to yield the greatest healing when you begin making it your own.

IT TAKES EFFORT TO BECOME EFFORTLESS

I don't want to make it sound like there's no learning curve involved. As we talked about in the previous chapter, The Method requires some patient practice as you start doing check-ins and tuning into your internal navigation system, especially during moments of heightened stimulus and stress.

As I always tell my clients, "It takes effort to become effortless." Most of us have learned this in one form or another. Maybe you were a natural athlete, but once you joined your high school team, your coach had to retrain you in the proper form. Maybe you were an early reader, but got certain pronunciations wrong until a teacher came along and corrected you. Natural aptitude almost always requires a few adjustments to help you get around certain resistances you didn't know you had.

There's no question that working with a coach trained in The Method can be extremely helpful. (If your navigation directs you toward that path, check out the Resources section at the end of the book for guidance on how to connect with our team and other services.) But be assured that any assistance we provide is directed toward helping you grow into your own sovereignty and Self-efficacy in a relatively short period of time.

You'll find that as soon as you get used to this new idea of becoming your own guide, healer, and leader of your life, your brain will immediately sense the improvement and start adapting to the change at lightning speed. It only takes a short time for your body, mind, and spirit to recognize how good it feels to connect to your true Self. Once that recognition takes place, the path for your life becomes even more practical, and you become even more inspired to increase your connection to your Self and live from that foundation. Being you and living life begins to feel effortless, the way it was always meant to be.

However, for people who genuinely want to live life to its fullest—healthy, happy, consciously connected to their purpose, and living their full potential—it's not the idea of effort that puts them off. What stands in their way, even when they believe The Method can help them, is the thought of going through it alone.

People will do just about anything if they believe it will contribute to their happiness. But maintaining that belief through the effort can be a real struggle, especially if you feel as if you're the only one doing what you're doing.

It's simply a fact that the process of healing singles you out from the crowd. Even when you're surrounded by people who are pursuing health, emotional well-being, or spiritual wholeness, the more time you spend with them, the more likely you are to discover that the majority are doing it for the wrong reasons. If you've ever been in a yoga class where it seems like everyone is trying to show off their skills, or joined a church only to find people judging each other, you know what I mean.

Community is an amazing resource, which is why I've shifted a lot of the work we do with clients to include a major component of community learning. But as you've learned by now, it's impossible to feel true connections with others until you first connect to your true Self. Without this connection, you will always feel lonely and unknown, even among the people closest to you.

For many people, learning to fully enjoy intimacy with the Self is the biggest shift involved in The Method. It feels unnatural to turn down an invitation without a "good excuse." As for making time to nurture themselves, some people feel so guilty about this that you'd think I'd directed them to spend their evening shouting insults at a box of newborn kittens.

But once you get past the awkward stage of spending quality time with your Self, you'll find your body and brain start reawakening in ways that will surprise you. You'll rediscover long-forgotten talents and become immersed in new passions. You'll find it getting easier and easier to schedule your time around the things you love without needing to find excuses for it. You'll start relishing the moments when you take your Self to dinner, plan a vacation with your Self, put your Self to bed at night. Before long, you'll be laughing at the thought of those years where you preferred spending holidays with your dysfunctional family or searching the Internet for a date over spending time with your Self.

The more closely you cultivate a good relationship with your Self, the more you'll realize that you've never been alone. Your Self has always been there, guiding you, comforting you, cheering you on as you navigate the world. Once you tune in to this connection with your Self, you fully and consciously feel how whole you are and always have been. You also become able to easily create the external connections and relationships you desire.

ACHIEVING REAL HAPPINESS

Maybe you're on the other end of the spectrum—you've been burned by so many relationships that you've given up looking for real connections, and the thought of community leaves a bad taste in your mouth. As far as you're concerned, people are just problems.

It's true that life without relationships might be a lot simpler. But be honest—would your life actually contain *more* joy if you had no relationships?

Again, it's not your relationships or the stress they can introduce that make you unhappy. It's not even the effort required to solve your stress. What makes you unhappy is believing that you're all alone in trying to solve your stress, that you're lost in a maze of issues with no real power to get back on the path to your potential.

Remember that pain, unfulfillment, and unhappiness are all fundamentally caused by not being in your potential. In contrast, real happiness comes when you are grounded in your Self, living your unique personal infrastructure, carving out your own path, and being confident in being your own advocate, your own guide, and your own best friend. Integrity with yourself is the highest experience of the evolutionary process, where each moment brings you into more of your potential. Once you have created this connection with your Self, it becomes easy to feel calm, confident, and capable when facing down the obstacles in front of you. It becomes intuitive to get blissfully absorbed in the activities that allow you to progress on the practical path to your purpose and potential.

And yes, your happiness is often amplified by sharing your full, complete Self with another person who is likewise whole and complete in themselves. Far from needing that person to "give" themselves to you, your commitment to your Self, and the way it brings about the most purposeful feeling of full potential, supports them in connecting more deeply with their own practical path.

By practicing The Method, you enjoy a day-to-day, moment-to-moment grounding in who you truly are and what your authentic purpose is. You never feel alone because you are fully experiencing the person who lives inside you. By learning to take care of your Self, you discover that you are your own greatest company.

This is where The Method switches from being a practice to a way of life. This is where you fall into the flow of effortless effort. Checking in with your Self, course correcting, applying your strength in one area to areas that need more development—this all becomes an effort in the same way that breathing is an effort or walking is an effort. You naturally keep doing it because it feels good. You have both the positive feelings of someone being interested in you, and the positive feelings of becoming deeply interested in someone...because both sides of the equation are actually you. All the while, going through The Method creates a feedback loop that makes connecting with your Self easier and more rewarding each time you do it.

Profound change doesn't happen overnight. It takes a while for The Method to work its way into every area of your life—health, job, family, romantic relationships, finances. It also takes time for the external adjustments you're making to stabilize, become automated within your Self, and grow more practical every day. However, taking your time is a good thing; making sudden, major shifts can be more harm than help. Like a shock to your system, it has the potential to leave you with a dissociative feeling that makes it difficult to recognize yourself.

Rather than jarring your system with sudden, seismic shifts, you're better off allowing your navigation to ease you into changes at a sustainable pace that allows those changes to be permanent. By surrendering to the slow evolution of The Method, you'll have the luxurious feeling of watching your true Self bloom.

MAKING THE METHOD YOUR OWN

No doubt you've experienced the frustration of having a friend, family member or even a therapist suggest you make a shift in your life that deep down, you know you aren't ready for. Maybe you've had someone sum up your issues with a way of thinking that you know isn't accurate. It does no good to argue—protesting against these voices only makes them more certain they are right.

Remember how in Chapter 4 we talked about a teacher's proper role in your life? You must bring that same principle into play when you start practicing The Method.

When you're in the midst of making unprecedented changes, it is easy and natural to solicit other people's feedback—*What do you think of the change in me? What pattern should I substitute for this old pattern I'm letting go? How should I go about getting the results I want to see?*

Allow me to set the record straight: *you* are the greatest living expert on your Self. Others' advice may be helpful in bringing up specific solutions you haven't thought of, but only your internal navigation system knows whether their ideas are useful in helping you live your purpose and potential.

Everybody who's fulfilled in a particular area of their

life usually thinks they have stumbled on the secret to happiness...and I'm not for a moment suggesting they haven't. However, the secret for them is not necessarily the secret for you.

The Method is simply a framework—you guide the process of applying it, and you decide how far to let it take you in each situation the day brings you. Thus, The Method belongs to anyone who chooses to use it. This means the way you practice The Method will be different from every other patient I've ever treated. The Method is not Dr. Tracy's Method. It is *your* Method.

TAKING CARE OF YOUR SELF = SERVING OTHERS

My husband and I are avid ballroom dancers. We take lessons every week and start nearly every morning with an hour of practice before breakfast. It's a really fun way to kick off our day by waking up our physical bodies, connecting with music and rhythm, and whirling in and out of each other's arms.

Ballroom dancing is based on the principle of lead and follow, which means each "move" or pattern of steps is initiated by one partner (the "lead") giving cues to the other (the "follow"), who can carry out the move with a variety of stylized flourishes. It demands a lot of trust between the partners, not to mention close physical communication.

In our dance partnership, my husband serves as the lead. But that doesn't mean our success as a couple depends on him. He has certain moves he's very good at leading and others that are challenging for him. If I want us to be the best dancers we can be, I have to hone my ability to feel and respond to his cues. The more I take care of my Self as a dancer by developing my ability to understand the information he gives me, the better I perform.

Of course, the reverse is also true. My husband could get fed up with my inability to follow cues that he is giving to the best of his current ability. But instead, he tries different ways of physically communicating the information about what move he's trying to lead.

The better each of us performs individually, the better we perform as a couple. Even in a dance that requires two partners, we are both best served when we take care of our own needs first. For this reason, we always start with personal practice for the first half of the morning before embarking on partner practice in the second half. It's essential to know your Self first so you can share that Self with the other, in dance as well as in life.

When you're trying to take care of everyone else in your life, all you're really doing is attempting to control your environment to ensure that your needs get met. But as you may have figured out by now, controlling your environment is an impossible task. When you stop trying to be superhuman and start paying attention to your own needs first, you'll find that not only are you happier, but other people in your life start to look after their own needs, as well. It's a simple system, but that's what makes it so practical *and* successful.

MEASURING YOUR PROGRESS WITH THE METHOD

In most forms of therapy, the patient waits for the therapist to let them know when they are "done." Some patients wait for this moment eagerly, while others live in dread of being released back "into the wild."

By now, it probably won't surprise you to learn that The Method doesn't work like that. When my team and I work with a patient, we aren't measuring their progress against the day when they are "fixed," because the whole premise is they were never broken to begin with. We are simply there to facilitate them on the journey of discovering their own true Self; and, in doing so, they find the simplicity and practicality of living their purpose and potential. It's not this super confusing thing that is meant to baffle and elude them.

If your navigation drives you to work with my team and me in one of our Live Your Potential Academy programs, then fabulous! Believe me, there's nothing I'd love more than to work with you directly in helping you incorporate The Method into your life in the most accelerated way possible. But I also want you to know that following The Method is just as effective when you practice it on your own.

A coach's main function is to help you see more clearly what your Self already knows. With or without a coach, your progress ultimately depends on you taking action—choosing to move forward with each practical step on the path your Self reveals to you.

Again, it's not the milestones or the majorly eventful before/after images that you're going for. It's an ever-closer connection with your internal navigation system, a more seamless alignment of your actions with your purpose and potential, and a continual building towards epic emotional strength.

Even though transformation happens at lightning speed compared to most other processes (this is flying direct rather than having a bunch of layovers), I advise people not to judge or evaluate the process until a year has gone by. Even though our clients experience immediate results, it's important not to let today's progress be derailed by your urgency for tomorrow's. Instead of looking at the "big picture"—the radical makeover of your entire life—focus on the "deep picture"—the way your internal landscape is shifting, healing, emerging. The more you invest your attention on the deep internal shifts of today, the more potential you'll have for making additional shifts tomorrow. You don't have to take my word for it—go to https://www.drtracyinc.com/testimonials/ where you can read client testimonials as well as listen to video interviews with clients who have shared firsthand the challenges they were struggling with prior to adopting The Method, and the positive transformation in their life as a result of The Method.

Within a few months of focusing on the internal adjustments, the external adjustments will begin to jump out at you. Your skin will start to glow, your sleep will improve, you'll become more formidable at your job, your relationships will cease to feel like a minefield. You'll find yourself catching your breath throughout the day—"Wow, is this really my life now?" The more you move your life in the direction of your practical path, the more you'll like the way your life looks... because it looks like you. At the one-year mark, you'll have gone through all four seasons of actioning your awareness, and you'll be in awe of what a difference one year makes.

For every adjustment you choose to make, allow your

internal navigation system to set the pace and intensity for you. For example, if you're trying to adopt a healthier lifestyle, let your internal navigation system guide you not only about which gym to join, but which classes to take, how long to spend on each machine, etc. If you need to level up (or down) for the day or for the month, let your internal navigation guide you there as well. And if you're about to go on that vacation to Italy you've dreamed about for years, trust your internal navigation system to guide you to the experience your Self genuinely desires. Why stay in the budget hotels if what you really want is a luxurious getaway in a private villa? Why wander around a city trying to feel appropriately awestruck about ancient art and architecture, if what you really want is an immersive experience in a tiny hilltop village? Don't take the trip everybody says you're supposed to have—create the adventure your Self truly desires.

Perhaps you've got several issues that you'd like to address. If that's the case, let your internal navigation system guide you in which ones to tackle right away and which ones to address at a later point on your path. Again, shocking your system by trying to adjust too much, too fast, is only going to delay your process, because your internal navigation system would never direct you to do something like that. Now that you know The Method, don't use it to bully, berate, or undermine your Self. The way you implement The Method is as important as The Method itself.

Remember, you are in charge of a precious human life—your own. The degree to which you love and care for your Self will set the precedent for how other people love and care for you. You will be shocked by how quickly the world offers you exactly what you desire when you care for your Self as your most precious resource. So, if you'd like to work directly with me and my team, go to thedrtsolution. com.

Chapter Ten

RELATING: EVERYTHING YOU ARE AND EVERYTHING YOU DO IS CONNECTED

No matter how often children are told "you're so special" by their parents, it's still very rare for them to truly connect with themselves and their unique purpose when they don't see their parents providing that example. The result is a vast cognitive disconnect that becomes glaringly obvious once the child grows up and begins forming relationships, especially the romantic kind.

As we dive into The Method's redesign of how to "do" relationships, let's start by reaffirming the fundamental truth that you were told, but never taught: you *are* unique. From your hair color to your height, from the way your body processes medication to what your brain does well (and not so well), to how all these factors affect your psychology, there is no exact genetic code like the one you carry inside of you. It is scientifically true that you are unique, unrepeatable, and you need customized Self-care.

But without knowing how to create a relationship with your Self, the feeling of uniqueness can translate in your psyche as a feeling of loneliness. Combined with a sense of lack and a disconnection from your Self, this feeling creates a subconscious drive to seek out relationships in the belief that someone else's love can finally meet all your needs, giving you that feeling of purpose and the experience of more potential. The more you've been hurt, the less productive your relationship choices become. You may form a relationship with someone who is negligent or abusive. Or, you may choose to "settle" for someone who doesn't really attract you. These are both sides of the same coin—lying to your Self out of desperation to experience "connection."

As we've talked about previously, this strategy is doomed to fail every time. It *is* connection you need, but not with someone else. You need to create the connection with your Self. And like it or not, your true Self is always demanding the very best for you in every aspect of your life. In fact, knowing and embracing your own uniqueness is essential in living your practical path.

Instead of trying to fulfill someone else's expectations while depending on them to satisfy your unique needs, you must learn to treat your Self as unique. That means giving your Self a unique and customized level of priority of your care. In addition to following your internal navigation system's leading in how you act in the world, you must also learn to be emotionally available to your Self in those moments where life doesn't turn out how you expected.

Nowhere is this more true than when it comes to love and sex—the "holy grail" of experiencing potential, where two people attempt to walk their paths together.

HOLLYWOOD ROMANCE, DECONSTRUCTED

The whole world is trying to figure out how to "do" love. In light of all the conflicting advice around romantic relationships (or maybe because of it), many people have tried to create an approach to love and romance that is a lot less, well, romantic. Ask someone for advice, and they're bound to say something like, "Love is hard work," or "Relationships are messy."

The only reason relationships are messy is because people approach them that way. Love is only hard work when you make it impractical through ignoring the needs of your true Self to such a degree that you cannot connect to your purpose or experience your full potential. In the same way that we go through life making everything a struggle simply by expecting it to be that way, we create problems in our relationships before they even get started by expecting them to be confusing, chaotic, and disappointing...*unless* we work really hard, in which case they'll offer us the "at last" sense of fulfillment we've been waiting for all our lives. You know, the "You complete me" bullshit that keeps Hollywood in business.

These polar extremes of disappointment/fulfillment, and the confusing struggle in between, is what makes romance such a popular subject for films. But what distinguishes a romantic comedy from a romantic drama is the tone in which the mess is approached. We can laugh with guiltless entertainment while watching the pitfalls of lovelorn characters when those characters come off as strong and resilient. But when the characters are demonstrably fragile, insecure, prone to Self-sabotage, then we watch with transfixed horror like spectators at the site of a freeway pileup.

These two tropes reveal a kernel of truth within the shallow Hollywood formula: a relationship with someone else can only be as strong as your relationship to your Self. If you've never had practice creating a loving relationship with your Self, you're setting your Self up for disappointment—maybe even disaster—by making a commitment to a partner, whether it be casual or lifelong. Instead of enjoying and appreciating your partner's Self, you're going to spend all your time together trying to meet their needs and trying to make them meet yours.

In my experience working with couples, I've found that most couples are drawn together by primal drives that connect to the best in each other. But because they do not know how to be in integrity with themselves while in a relationship, they find it impossible to experience the level of potential they desire the relationship to have or be, while becoming romantically involved with someone. They believe that successful relationships mean that both partners live the same path. They don't realize that this is impractical in the short-term and unsustainable in the long run.

IT ALL COMES BACK TO YOU

Look back on your relationships—the ones that blew up in your face no matter how hard you tried to make them work, the ones you wanted but never got the chance to explore, the ones that worked pretty well but never brought the sense of bliss or completeness you expected. What would you say is the common denominator among all your relationships?

Got your answer? Okay. Now kick it to the curb, because it's wrong.

I don't care if you said it was "looking for a father figure" or "being attracted to abusers" or "someone put me on a pedestal" or anything else.

The real common denominator is *you.*

All your relationships with others are mirrors of how you relate to your Self. Dig deeply into the nature of the conflicts you've had with your significant others, and I guarantee that you'll find a version of the same fight you have with your Self. Moreover, the ways your significant other "fails" your expectations are all reflections of the lack inside you.

One classic way this plays out is the savior model of relationship, where one person's pity for another person's problems becomes a romantic crusade to save them from themselves. If you haven't done this yourself, you've probably watched a friend do it. Alternatively, maybe you've experienced it from the side of the person who needs saving.

Both sides of the relationship are ultimately coming from the same place—they are both looking to the other person to supply their lack of purpose and direction, to complete the Self.

I talk constantly with clients who are befuddled by the way they seem to repeatedly end up in "messiah" relationships with partners who seem to pull away the more they are trying to "save" or "help," and seem uninterested in committing or caring at the level they desire. As the client describes the ins and outs of the relationship to me, I wait for the point when I can help them realize they were getting out of these relationships exactly the relationship they have with themselves. While they believed they were investing love, patience, help, and wisdom into this other person, what they were really investing was a Self trying to outsource those things from someone else. Is it any wonder that the person they were trying to love decided to look elsewhere? The same goes if you're the person in the relationship that is trying to be made over.

Both parties are trying to get or do something for some-one that they need to look to themselves for. This is my definition of insanity.

ALL'S FAIR IN LOVE AND WAR

If you're like a lot of people, love and war may feel like one and the same to you by this time. In other words, many people treat love like a form of rivalry, bringing their best strategy, scheming, and emotional weaponry to the battlefield. (No 1980s pop song pun intended.) You may have reached the point where you don't even feel like you're in a relationship unless every interaction has a clear winner and loser.

If this is where you're at, I have to break it to you: you're not in love. You're in a war. And the war isn't with your significant other. It's with your Self. Your lover is simply a proxy for the failures, the weaknesses, and the flaws you see in your Self.

You may protest, "No, my partner couldn't be more dif-ferent from me; he/she is strong in all the ways I'm not." Choosing someone who explicitly embodies your flaws and weaknesses is entry-level stuff. You may have made the most mature choice for a romantic partner that you've ever made in your life, and found someone who is balanced and healthy. These are the very situations that people find the most maddening—they believe they've fixed their romantic pathologies and are enjoying the healthiest relationship of their lives, yet they're still having ongoing conflicts with their partner. Their attempts to resolve these conflicts are seldom productive. They live in a state of terminal disappointment.

The reason is simple: if you don't settle the war with your Self first, you will constantly be at war with your romantic partner.

Obviously, some relationships simply do not fit with being in integrity with your Self.

If you're in a relationship that subjects you to personal harm, you need to leave that relationship—end of story. But let's talk in this chapter about how to stay in a good relationship and make it better.

RETHINKING "WORK" IN RELATIONSHIPS

I have served as a consultant and contributor to countless "love advice" columns in national magazines. I always laugh when I'm asked my opinion for yet another "how to make him or her do this, that, or the other" article. These writers know by now that no matter how the question is reiterated, my answer will always come back to the same principle: *Whatever you want your partner to be, become that yourself.*

The "hard work" in relationships is nothing more than trying to make someone else be what you want them to be. You know, someone that makes you complete, that brings out your "best Self."

In reality, that's not hard work—that's an impossible task.

No matter how you define a successful love life—a lifelong marriage or a series of satisfying short-term relationships, a deep emotional friendship or just a regular helping of good sex—it will be out of your reach until you create a successful relationship with your Self.

Next time you begin listing all the qualities you'd need in your ideal partner, look at the person you're designing and ask your Self if such a person would want to date you. The fact is that you can't design your ideal partner, and you definitely can't make your ideal person want to be with you or perform the way you expect in a relationship. The only life you have that kind of control over is your own. This makes it your obligation to prioritize the evolution of your Self into its highest form so it can exist in all aspects of your life—as a higher being creating a higher experience with no limits. This is your purpose here on Earth, and this is what potential is all about.

This goes against almost everything we are taught. The popular definition of love is being willing, even glad, to sacrifice your own needs and desires for the good of someone else.

I'll acknowledge that some of the most personally fulfilling moments of my marriage have involved making a choice to spend my effort or time on behalf of my husband's happiness. However, the reason I'm able to make those choices at all is because I've had a lot of practice making them on behalf of my Self.

Just as we talked about in Chapter 6, choosing the long-term best for your Self means sacrificing the immediate desires and impulses in any given moment in exchange for more potential in the long-term. I've adjusted my taste for pleasure in favor of a good that goes deeper than any instant gratification. In doing so, I enjoy an even more instantaneous gratification—that of nourishing my Self at the most foundational level.

At this point, my Self-fulness has grown so abundantly that it naturally spills over into my relationship with my husband. As a result, none of my choices on his behalf feel like sacrifice—they feel as natural as anything my Self might do for me.

Finally, practicing Self-fulness protects me from watering down the choices I make for him with an expectation that he do the same for me. Nothing takes the delight out of a gift like realizing the giver is expecting something from you in return...or, worse yet, is waiting for you to read their mind and know what they expect from you. If I have already given my Self everything it needs to feel loved, nourished, and cared for, then anything my husband does for me (and he does a lot!) is just overabundance.

Saying "love is work" is looking at relationships from the wrong angle. I'd say that love is overabundance added to overabundance—two people sharing with each other out of an overflowing fulfillment of their unique Selves, creates a sense of purpose and a fulfillment of potential.

The best part is that, in doing this, we give each other not only the excess of our own abundance, but we also give each other the freedom to continue growing and progressing on our unique paths. My husband and I both recognize that in wanting the other one to be happy, the best thing we can give each other is an empowering free-dom to meet our own needs. Sometimes this is done in partnership, as in our ballroom dancing endeavors. Other times, this is done separately. Sometimes I go to a party while he stays at home, and sometimes he's going out while I'm staying home. Sometimes one of us will agree to adjust our individual plans to prioritize spending time together. But these are things we do only when we have sufficiently met our own needs and filled ourselves with so much Self-love that we have plenty to share. Whether together or apart, we help each other connect with our fullest potential in each moment.

I love the moment when our "couple clients" get this concept. They look at each other with new eyes—not as enemies, but as team members. Love, like life, is just not meant to be complicated. It delivers so much more of the bliss we desire when we let it be practical.

RECALIBRATING YOUR ROMANCE

It can be difficult to start focusing on your Self when your relationship is in a challenging place. Even if you can embrace the idea of cultivating a good relationship with your Self as a foundation to heal what's broken in your love life, you may find that other people are less confident about the result of your efforts. Your significant other may be resentful. Your friends may be skeptical. Your parents will almost certainly have something to say about it.

These objections are good signs. They are proof that you're departing from the normal standard of relationships...and isn't following the normal standard exactly what got you to the trouble you're in?

Don't feel obligated to explain to others what you're doing or why it's important. Trying to get other people's understanding or affirmation of your commitment to your Self is usually a waste of energy. As in all other aspects of following the path to your purpose and potential, living it is much more powerful than explaining it.

If doubts arise in your own mind, remember that working on your relationship with your Self *is* working on the relationship with your partner. Without recalibrating your own connection to your Self on an ongoing basis, you'll never achieve the potential for a deep (albeit practically accomplished) connection with another person. Doing so would be like trying to tune a beat-up guitar to a warped old piano. All it accomplishes is making two instruments play off-key.

A relationship gets out of tune because each partner goes into it expecting the other person to know them, understand them, and give them meaning. They only give as much as they believe they can, and then get frustrated when they're not getting back as much as they feel they deserve. Doesn't it make sense that if each of us focused on fulfilling our own needs and the experience of full potential, we would have so much more to give?

What you're expecting from others is something you can only give your Self. The sooner you realize that, the sooner you'll be prepared to experience the true love you've always yearned for.

LIVING IN INTEGRITY—THE SECRET INGREDIENT

Like everything else, relationships must be lived in integrity with your Self. Each partner must be committed to each other's individual pursuit of fulfillment, and be ready to support that process without controlling, judging, or being in fear of it.

Obviously, there are some relationships that will not survive under this model. The most out-of-integrity relationships are marked by extreme imbalance between the partners, along with a severe limitation of one or both people's freedom. If the only things that attract you to another person are their pathologies, their brokenness, their weakness, and need, then the relationship is probably going to dissolve as soon as one or both of you learns to live in integrity with yourselves.

However, in my experience, most relationships *can* be

salvaged when each partner commits to refocusing their priorities around their relationship to themselves. It's not unusual that when your partner sees you on the path to your own purpose and potential, they feel drawn to follow their own path, as well.

When you take away the codependence, the misconceptions about love, and the habituated patterns, you're left with a couple of people who are still attracted to the best in each other. Add in a supreme confidence that flows from genuine well-being and you've got the potential for some hot and heavy romance. There's nothing more exciting than two people who are attracted to each other sharing the potential to help each other follow their own paths.

CHANGING THE WAY YOU LOOK

Most people go into a romantic relationship trying to fix the way they look—they cut their hair, they work on their abs, they buy a new wardrobe. If they're really trying to make a change, they may practice standing with better posture, learn some jokes or trivia facts, or study techniques on using body language, all in an effort to look more confident, more humorous, more intellectual, and more attractive.

Compare that approach to the statement by physicist Max

Planck, "When you change the way you look at things, the things you look at change."

This is exactly what The Method asks of you. Changing your appearance and demeanor isn't really about how you appear to others; it's an attempt to appear more worthy of love to your Self. However, when you come into a relationship seeing your Self as being in need of someone else to fulfill your purpose or complete your potential, you're setting the other person up to let you down.

Even if you reached the apex of sexiness as you define it, and even if you get into bed every night with the most attractive partner you could ever dream of, you will always be looking for something more because you fundamentally fail to experience fulfilling connection with your own potential. Moreover, you will never give that partner the love and attention they desire because you will be looking at them through the same lens you use to look at your Self.

By contrast, once you start to look at your Self with love, satisfaction, admiration, and respect, you will start seeing the people around you in the same way. Your dating life will transform from a litany of disappointments to a landscape of intriguing possibilities. Your marriage will stop feeling like a habit you can't shake and turn into a deep, soul-enriching, side-by-side adventure.

Perhaps you don't need any help in the romance department. Perhaps your relationship is the brightest spot in your life and your partner encourages you in seeking fulfillment of your purpose and potential. Perhaps you're content being single and have no desire to seek love outside of your family and friends.

I would still venture that you have at least one relationship in your life that could use a new look. Maybe it's not even a relationship to a person. Maybe instead, it's your relationship to food, or money, or creativity.

See how we've come back to where we started?

The idea that our lives are fractured into discrete sections—health, career, money, family, love life—is a complete fallacy. All of these aspects are parts of one whole, which means that any success in one area begets success in the others. Living in integrity with your Self means knitting together your entire life with a unified purpose. It means consistent attunement to the internal navigation system. It means constant, loving advocacy for your Self and a greater feeling of purpose and potential in every moment.

Think back to Chapter 7, where we talked about building

the matrix. Every improvement you make in your relationships will create a pattern for the same improvement in your career, your health, and everywhere else. Some people choose to focus a little bit on each area of their life in turn, while others choose to concentrate on applying The Method to one area for some time, then move on to another area. It's really up to you to decide what your internal navigation is drawing you toward. There's no bad decision when it comes to creating your unique path, as long as each step is practical.

Furthermore, applying The Method also has the power to transform bad decisions in your past. It's easy to look back and regret mistakes, especially when it comes to relationships. However, living in integrity with your Self asks that you love, honor, and have compassion for the person who made those past decisions. After all, we'd all do better if we knew better.

You can't erase the past, nor should you. The experiences you've had of feeling lost, confused, or left behind, even if painful, are valuable R&D hours logged in pursuit of who you really are and what kind of relationships do and don't work for you. With The Method, you don't have to disown those decisions or the person who made them. Instead, you can move forward with confidence and purpose, understanding what the lessons of the past have taught you, and teaching your Self to receive the gift of unconditional acceptance and grace. This book serves as the foundational launching pad to achieve this goal.

If you'd like to comprehensively upgrade the relationship with your Self as well as every relationship in your life, our online emotional strength training programs can take you to the next level. Go to thedrtsolution.com to learn more.

CONCLUSION

———

"This above all: to thine own self be true
And it must follow, as the night the day
Thou canst not then be false to any man."
—*HAMLET*, ACT I, SCENE III

Maybe being true to your Self was an easy matter in Shakespeare's time. In today's world, it can be a lot more complicated. We feel pulled in hundreds of different directions by people who insist we find personal fulfillment in fulfilling *their* agenda. We allow ourselves to be inundated by technology that is supposed to give us more time, but ends up taking it away from us. We're willing to digest an ever-changing array of messages from the media on what is beautiful, what is true, and what is meaningful.

We make living our purpose and potential a mysterious, laborious endeavor.

The challenge isn't just putting all these elements together into a whole. It's feeling as though you're in a fishbowl, being watched by everyone in your life and judged for the choices you make.

Living in the world means living under the gaze of other people. It's as much a part of our milieu as living under a sky, within a blanket of oxygen. But when you choose to live from the connection to your Self and to action your awarenesses, you feel a sense of purpose in everything you do and a fulfillment of potential. As a result, your life is a transforming force for the lives of everyone around you.

BE YOUR POTENTIAL

The world has this idea that real change doesn't happen without huge personal sacrifice or heroic efforts. Most people look at figures like Rosa Parks, Nelson Mandela, or Mother Teresa and think, "Now *there's* a life that matters." What we never realize is that for those people, the sacrifice came well before their heroic actions. The transformative things they did were nothing more than practical steps on the path of their purpose and living a life of potential.

When you come right down to it, most heroic actions are fairly simple—performing a kind act, voicing your opinion, standing up or even keeping your seat on a bus. What makes those actions revolutionary is doing them outside of the parameters other people have deemed acceptable. When you realize that your choice is between existing in social comfort, which was never that comfortable anyway, and being comfortable in your own Self, you'll find that it's surprisingly easy to be a hero.

As you begin to act in integrity, you'll be shocked at how un-sacrificial it feels. Quite the contrary—it feels like a luxury. What starts as saying no to attending a party could end up, in a year from now (or less!), as traveling the world to bring medicine to the indigent, or composing a symphony, or completing your yoga teacher training. It could be as simple as inspiring someone else with your story, who then goes on to transform their own life.

Living in integrity with your Self is what allows you to live in integrity with the rest of the world. Every action you take that is truthful, respectful, and loving toward your Self brings the people around you that much closer to connecting with their own purpose and living their potential.

Your life matters. Your purpose and potential has immense significance for the good of this planet, and those who are living their full potential make the greatest positive impact of all. Think of all the people who have followed their sense of purpose and passion for what they feel they must bring to our world, and how that literally changes the way we live.

Your ability to live your purpose and fulfill your potential matters more than anything. You'll never know how much until you start living it.

TIME TO GO TO WORK

As much as I'd like to take credit for "inventing" The Method, it was really much simpler than that. The Method is nothing less than my true Self living its purpose and potential, connecting to others doing the same. The combined forces of our true Selves are the greatest universal forces that exist. We simply need to have the courage to live by it, rather than wait until we feel we have no choice.

Just like me, you have always known that there was a Self inside you, filled with purpose and potential, ready and waiting to make its mark. You've now reached a point, just like I did, where you can't ignore it anymore.

Your path is waiting for you. Now is your moment to move forward.

As you embrace and implement the tenants of The Method and experience true epic emotional transformation, keep in mind that you also have an opportunity to take your Self to the next level by joining a community of people learning and applying the Method into their life every day. Join Our Free Facebook Group—The Art of Self Control.

I have provided a list of resources in More Things to Help You. Further, if you'd like to comprehensively upgrade the relationship with your Self as well as every relationship in your life, our online emotional strength training programs can take you to the next level. Go to thedrtsolution.com to learn more.

ACKNOWLEDGMENTS

———

This book has been a lifetime in the making, with countless experiences, trials, and errors, and the dedication to grow into the highest version of myself possible—all of these allowing me to better serve those suffering to live in their greatest potential. Yet, it wouldn't have been possible had it not been for the many people with whom I've shared my life:

The teams of people I've trained have taught me so much. As a result of the opportunities to lead and manage, I've been able to not only hone these skills, but see what it means to bring out the best in people.

The gifts given by my clients each day cannot be overstated. I'm inspired by their dedication, commitment, and perseverance in applying The Method. Humbled by their investment, willingness, openness, courage, and trust (and that of their families as well). Honored to partner with them in transforming their lives out of the depths of hell and into a sense of self-containment, self-mastery, and security. Not only am I privileged to witness their tenacity in carving out their personal path of purpose and potential, I'm also motivated by their example to refine and expand The Method, so that all who choose to employ it can do so on every level and in every detail.

The bedrock of this book is solidified by my mom's unconditional love and support, which has been there for me my entire life, along with her great recognition of my highest self and my pure potential. Seeing through my "Mommy's" eyes has allowed me to recognize the best of who I am, which has helped me through dark and confusing moments—moments when I mistakenly believed I was something or someone other than my highest Self. The work I do would not be possible without the compassion my mom passed on to me. Thank you, Mom, and thank you to my stepdad, Duane, for always having my back.

This book wouldn't have happened without everything that my father modeled for me about being an entrepreneur. His lessons in self-determination forged my business acumen, my athletic-conditioning mentality, and my tenacity. These skills allowed me to combine the strengths of a top business person with the acumen and training of a transformative leader in the field of clinical psychology. These key ingredients helped me develop a structured methodology that changes lives on a level that is not only metaphysical, but practical, logistical, and lasting. Thank you, Dad, for showing me what it means to develop self-mastery and excellence in these areas of life.

The struggles my family has been through formed the foundation for this book. I acknowledge all my family members for their survival and their courage, and for the fun we've had together through it all. They taught me that life isn't just about getting by; it's amusing, entertaining, hilarious—and when it comes right down to it, laughter in life is a must. This has become a hallmark of my methodology and I have them to thank for it.

I am so thankful for the romantic partners who have been in my life. They gave me the opportunity to see my true Self as we worked on growing our relationships together. Because of them, I was able to identify what doesn't work and what causes pain, which helped me uncover the real meaning of connection, love, and evolution. They showed me that being able to grow together means growing while you're together. Thank you for learning how to be a person alongside me, and for trying to be the person I needed while I was learning that the person I'd been waiting for was me.

Professionally, where I am today would not have been possible without Dr. Adriana Popescu. She gave me my first counseling internship, which brought my first opportunities in the field of addiction and therapeutic treatment. Adriana's ability to see what I was and who I was, and her willingness to offer me the latitude to run with my own my method and develop it into The Method, made her the right mentor at the right time. And that, as the poem says, has made all the difference.

Alta Mira Recovery is where I made the biggest strides in testing the principle that came to be the foundation for The Method and for this book. Without the opportunity to work with this group—to see what it's like to use this methodology with people who can afford anything—I would never have witnessed The Method's full potential. It's ability to change lives and entire family legacies. The leadership role I was given at Alta Mira was truly career-making on a foundational level.

This book also exists because of the extraordinary and unconditional love, support, and encouragement of my girlfriends:

The friends who've been with me since kindergarten have always given me the freedom to be me...starting with allowing me to entertain them since we were all five years old. (My original therapeutic modality!) These friends have always accepted the me that I am and encouraged me to do me...even when I'm off fulfilling my purpose in work (or in play). Their encouragement has meant the world to me during the writing of this book and through building this business.

My friends from New York have allowed me to be the group therapist as we navigated our lives in true "Sex and the City" fashion. As true supporters, they've always told me how smart, intuitive, and great I am at helping people solve problems, feel better, and figure themselves out. By showing trust and faith in the advice I gave them, they enabled me to become the coach I am today. Thanks to their encouragement to follow my path, I'm able to live the purpose they clearly identified in me.

Not only would this book not have been possible without the teachers I've learned so much from—Oprah Winfrey, Byron Katie, Marianne Williamson, Eckhart Tolle, Brené Brown, Tony Robbins, Adyashanti, and others—but I might not even be here. My particular thanks goes to Oprah, the original therapist and teacher. Her show gave me a path for becoming my best Self.

Thank you to my team at Dr. Tracy Inc. for making this possible and for picking up the slack while I wrote this book. I am in awe of how they brilliantly carry out this methodology every day with our clients—the first step in making it possible for people to heal, recover, and live to their fullest potential. I am immensely grateful for their courage in living this method no matter how difficult, for showing integrity with clients, and for all of their love and support.

These people changed their lives to be able to work with me, placing their trust in me as they carry out my directions. The only greater privilege than being their boss is serving as their mentor.

To Carla and some of my clients, I'm considered a mentor—a privilege I am deeply conscious of. Without Carla, I would never have had the system to make this book a reality. My sincere thanks to her for connecting me with Lion's Head Publishing.

I also want to give special acknowledgment to Kristen. She learned the methodology by working for me and took it to heart in every way. Her unique ability to understand me has made for a wonderful collaboration, allowing me to build a more extensive business so more people are able to receive The Method more efficiently. Kristen brings The Method to life, reflects it back to me, and brings it to our clients on a world-class level. Every day. She puts the methodology into every aspect of Dr. Tracy Inc., and has dedicated herself fully to this methodology. She is the conscious collaborator that I'd been waiting for.

Big thanks to my publishing team at Lioncrest—Chelsea, Elizabeth, Tom, and Ellie. There is no better crew when you need help saying what you want to say and getting out of your own way. Their leadership and guidance has made a lifelong dream possible.

I want to acknowledge my colleagues who collaborate in doing this work with me. They have taught me so much about human health and well-being and have made possible the holistic healing I facilitate for my clients.

Enormous thanks to all my dance teachers for showing me so much about being a person and helping me grow in relationship with myself. There are some things you just can't learn by listening and reading; you have to learn them through your body with the help of somebody else's wisdom. These teachers make me want to learn more, grow more, and share more.

To my husband, Bruce, about whom there are so many things I could say. Since we met and fell in love, Bruce has been with me every step of the way, in everything. I am eternally grateful for his unconditional love, for his unwavering support and dedication, for his ability to see our marriage as something greater than the struggle of one person or another, for his commitment to the vision for our life and our business, and for living that out together.

When I met my husband, it was the ultimate affirmation that The Method not only works, but that it works beyond anything that I could ever have fathomed. Our relationship is the greatest partnership of my life and teaches me more about my Self than anything ever has.

Bruce has been with me in every detail of this book and every part of this process. He was the driving force behind so many aspects of this book and the relationship with the publisher. Doing all this life/business with someone who is the right Self for my Self was the final fulfilling part of making my life feel complete. It is because of him that I desire to be more of my highest Self and live more of my potential every day.

Thanks to TJ and Lola, my wiener dogs, who are a source of great motivation. I'm thankful to be able to continue to provide them with the life they've become accustomed to.

Finally, all my gratitude to my Grandma Bernice (Grammy). Along with my mother, she taught me what unconditional love is—to be totally adored. Knowing what that feels like allowed me to create the methodology of unconditionally loving yourself. I wouldn't have been able to bring humor to my life or this book without my grandmother and her wit. It was from her that I learned the importance of laughter, no matter how dark, treacherous, or traumatizing a situation may be. Her example taught me that if therapy is going to work, it has got to be fun.

In truth, my grandmother was my very first client. I grew up listening to her struggles, but also seeing her strive to live a life of integrity and doing things just because she wanted to. "I want to go to Hawaii—let's go. I want to go to dinner—let's go. I want to buy a piece of jewelry—I'm going to buy it." She gave me the first clue that the key to life lies in truly listening to yourself and taking action on what you know to be true. Through all her stress and struggle, she knew how to laugh and have fun. It was like she had a secret she was keeping just behind those dazzling eyes—a secret about how to make even the most difficult moments in life fun and full of potential.

ABOUT THE AUTHOR

—

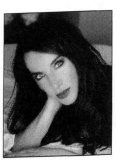 As the founder and first client of The Method, **DR. TRACY THOMAS** specializes in guiding people through their personal transformations. She is known not only for the speed and sustainability of her therapeutic coaching programs, but also for the energy, provocation, and comic relief that characterizes her approach.

Dr. Tracy's background includes a Ph.D. in psychology, master of arts in organizational development, and bachelor of arts in business management, with over twenty years of experience coaching, teaching, consulting, and serving as an expert resource to various journalists and over twenty national media outlets and publications.

Having trained numerous colleagues in her cognitive behavioral transformation and clinical life coaching techniques to become Dr. Tracy Certified Coaches, she now spends the bulk of her time developing courses, digital products, and other Self-guided content that equips individuals, couples, groups, and families with the internal resources to lead lives with intuition and intention.

When she isn't leading her team or guiding her clients through powerful training sessions, Dr. Tracy lives, works, and practices for her next ballroom-dancing championship in Northern California.

Made in the USA
Columbia, SC
06 October 2020